So It's Cancer: Now What?

Dr Ranjana Srivastava is a medical oncologist, Fulbright scholar, award-winning author and a columnist for *The Guardian*. After an upbringing in Bihar, India, and the United States, she graduated from Monash University in Melbourne, Australia, with first-class honours. Ranjana is the winner of the Monash University Distinguished Alumni award and practices in the Australian public hospital system.

Ranjana has written widely on the subject of medicine and humanity and ethics. She publishes frequently in the *New England Journal of Medicine* and her work has also appeared in *The Lancet*, *JAMA*, *Annals of Internal Medicine*, *Time*, *The Week*, *The Age* and several other publications including *Australia's Best Science Writing*. She has won the Cancer Council Victoria award for outstanding writing as well as the Gus Nossal Prize for Global Health writing.

Her first book, *Tell Me the Truth: Conversations with My Patients about Life and Death*, was short listed for a major literary award. Her second book, *Dying for a Chat: The Communication Breakdown Between Doctors and Patients*, won the Australian Human Rights Commission Literature Prize. Ranjana's interest in explaining and demystifying medicine to the general public has led to a regular presence on the Australian Broadcasting Corporation network. Her roles as a medical volunteer have included working with the Asylum Seeker Resource Centre in Melbourne, with the Missionaries of Charity in Calcutta and in post-tsunami Maldives.

Ranjana lives in Melbourne with her family.

So It's Cancer: Now What?

RANJANA SRIVASTAVA

HARPER
element

First published in 2014 by Penguin Books, Australia

First published in India in 2015 by Harper Element
An imprint of HarperCollins *Publishers*

Building 10, Tower A, 4th Floor, DLF Cyber City, Phase II,
Gurugram Haryana – 122002, India
www.harpercollins.co.in

P-ISBN: 978-93-5177-112-8
E-ISBN: 978-93-5177-113-5

2 4 6 8 10 9 7 5 3 1

Typeset in 10.5/13.5 Electra LT Std
By Saanvi Graphics Noida

Printed and bound at
MicroPrints India, New Delhi

For Swati and the gift of friendship

'If you have one true friend, you have more than your share.'

– Thomas Fuller

Contents

Foreword

It gives me great pleasure to write a foreword to *So It's Cancer: Now What?* by Dr Ranjana Srivastava. The book has been a great eye-opener for me. Having been involved with oncology and clinical work over the last thirty years, I too have gone through most of the experiences that she has described in her work as an oncologist. However, the way Ranjana has translated her knowledge and experience into simple and beautiful prose is original and unique.

I believe that being a physician is itself a great privilege, a gift of God, as it allows him or her to delve into the most intricate and beautiful mechanisms of life. But being a medical oncologist is a greater privilege. Oncology has emerged as the most comprehensive medical science, one that brings the healer spiritually and socially very close to those who are suffering over long periods of time. It thus allows insight not only into the physical but also the mental health of a patient. Although great advances have been made in cancer science with dramatic outcomes particularly in childhood and many adult cancers, in cases like breast cancer and chronic myeloid leukaemia, cancer has become a chronic disease like diabetes. Simply prolonging life in many cancer patients has created new challenges.

Although set in Australia, this book will, without doubt, greatly support and inspire cancer patients in India, providing them invaluable information. Ranjana has virtually covered all aspects of experiencing cancer, and her writing will be of immense value to those affected as well as their caregivers, and help them to cope better. The book is quite detailed, and those with time will benefit by going through everything these pages offer. This is information very hard to obtain from busy doctors strapped for time.

Apart from giving the broad picture, Ranjana goes into fine and crucial detail, sharing things and answering questions that a patient may not even know he or she has! Clear answers have been provided to many questions that can arise from time to time during the treatment. Ranjana's writing is so accessible also because she describes her own experiences and personal anecdotes. For me, the most impressive chapters are on getting worse, managing pain, whether the oncologist has feelings, how long does a patient have, and if death will be painful.

Since the book has been written in a foreign setting, the Indian reader may perceive certain differences, for instance, occasional cultural differences. For example, patients and families in India may prefer a less direct form of communication with doctors while dealing with bad news and death. Such issues will require a more 'local' handling and approach.

But this in no way deters from the real and profound significance of *So It's Cancer, Now What?*. I highly commend this book, and I am sure it will impact millions of people in India. I also wish that it be made available in as many Indian languages as possible.

Dr Vinod Raina,
Director and Head, Department of Medical Haematology,
Haematology and Stem Cell Transplantation,
Fortis Memorial Research Institute, Gurgaon, India
(Formerly Professor and Head of Medical Oncology Institute
Rotary Cancer Hospital, All India Institute of Medical Sciences)
April 2015

Introduction

So you have been diagnosed with cancer. If the news is recent, your mind is probably still reeling from it. My patients often say that once they heard the word 'cancer', every other piece of information just evaporated – everything else said seemed like a tide of white noise. A common initial response is to feel upset that the diagnosis took time. You may be blaming yourself for not bringing it to attention earlier or annoyed that your concerns were ignored for too long. But sometimes there is just relief that finally someone has found the problem which can now be tackled.

The initial conversation around the disclosure of cancer is important. Being told the diagnosis in a frantic emergency department or in a theatre recovery room can be deeply unsettling and doesn't give you the opportunity to ask questions. People under the fog of an anaesthetic or in severe pain would find it almost impossible to concentrate on a serious conversation. Perhaps you learnt the diagnosis from your general practitioner (GP) who had hinted that he was worried about your weight loss.

If you have just met an oncologist you may have thought you were prepared to have a full discussion, but you turned into a mass of nerves no sooner you walked into the oncologist's office. Patients have apologized to me for crying in my room when they know that they should be spending that time understanding their diagnosis. Of course, they couldn't help but be upset or numbed by their circumstances.

These days there is such a wide range of available tests that it's not rare to find yourself in a situation where you are repeatedly told that although cancer is highly suspected you need to wait for a few more confirmatory tests. In that case, the remaining scans or biopsy, the surgery or the doctor's appointment can't come soon enough. Patients describe undergoing many tests but feeling starved for information and unable to start planning ahead. Are you one of them?

No matter where you are on the journey, feelings of fear, uncertainty, frustration and sadness are common. Patients are unsure about whom they can turn to. You may be surrounded by people dear to you but you are not quite sure how much to share and with whom. Is it better if everyone knows whatever you have been told, or will you slowly measure out the information? It's hard to gauge how much to make public and at what cost.

And above all, dealing with these countless new questions, you are probably asking yourself, why me, why now, what will happen ...? The rational side of you knows that cancer can happen to anyone but you can't help wondering why it's you and how you will cope. Different aspects of these emotions will strike you at different times. Sometimes you will feel vulnerable and other times in control of the situation. You may know or have been reassured that there has been great progress made in cancer treatment over the last decade, but how does this progress affect you? How will you navigate the journey ahead?

If being a cancer patient is challenging, being a family member or a close friend of a cancer patient can be just as challenging. What's more, it's a role that involves a great deal of internalization and silent worrying. You dearly want to help but are not sure how. Sometimes it feels right to respect a person's space but other times you suspect that the patient wants to talk but you have no idea how to broach a conversation. You are cautious not to upset feelings or make a bad situation worse with a careless remark.

The good news is that not everyone who is diagnosed with cancer faces a dire prognosis. Indeed, as treatments for common cancers improve, more and more people are alive to tell the story of their survival. Many people return to productive and satisfied lives although the story of survival is not always one of triumph. Survivors battle long-term anxiety, depression, body-image issues, and of course, the ever-present issue of recurrence that can overshadow even minor and reversible illness.

Whether you are a cancer patient, a family member or a survivor, you will know that the mere mention of cancer brings forth a wellspring of complex emotions. It might feel that all these questions are unique to you, because what you are going through no one else has or will in quite the same way. While every experience of cancer may be slightly different, what all those who come into contact with cancer do have in common is the wish to live a good life. Though you recognize that adjustments will have to be made, you want life with cancer to comprise more than a rolling series of tests, scans and doctors' appointments interspersed with worry. The keen gardener in you wants to keep gardening, the golfer still wants to smell the green, and the avid reader wants to keep up the attendance in his book club. You want to be well to attend family functions and entertain friends. When things go well, you want the ability to relish them. And in troubled times you still want to make the best out of your situation. Unlike a bout of appendicitis or a heart attack, cancer is not a discrete and episodic problem. And although survival rates have improved greatly in the past few decades, the diagnosis still overtakes and dramatically changes the rest of your life.

I am also thinking that as you read this you might be wondering who I am and how I am placed to offer you advice. The opportunity to accompany patients through a difficult time in their lives and form a relationship of trust with them appealed to me from an early age. I always yearned for continuity of care for my patients, meaning that I wanted a role in diagnosis, treatment and follow-up. My work as an oncologist has allowed me a privileged insight into all aspects of the experiences of cancer patients. Training in medical ethics and communication skills has given me another valuable perspective on how patients think. Since the publication of my first two books, I have been invited to talk with many patients, professionals, community and industry groups about cancer and all its human implications. I feel richly rewarded by these interactions because they have given me a very broad view of what really matters to patients.

Having shared their happiness and disappointment, their wonder and concern, I have thought for several years that all patients could do with plain language advice, provided with empathy and compassion, on navigating their new world. Having been a part of my patients' victories and challenges, I want to use what I now know to help you deal with your diagnosis. I want to help you make good decisions and also to sidestep some challenges.

There are two kinds of challenges cancer patients face. One is tackling the day-to-day mechanics of having cancer, such as making chemotherapy choices, keeping your weight stable or managing the side effects of treatment. It is understandably easy to become so absorbed by these issues that the big picture fades from attention. The big picture is about your aspirations, your goals of care in the context of the severity of your illness, knowing how to move forward as a survivor and, if indeed life is limited, how best to spend the remaining days. In my experience, for far too many people, the big picture comes into focus too late. I will confess here that part of this has to do with the way doctors communicate, with their focus too often also being on the immediate problems a patient faces. To use a firefighting analogy, while putting out spot fires might work elsewhere in medicine, cancer management is different. How one extinguishes a cancer spot fire is greatly determined by having an idea of the conflagration.

Unless you are medically trained it may be difficult to comprehend the pathology report or appreciate the changes on a computerized tomography (CT) scan, but the patients who navigate the journey well are those who always try to understand themselves and their motivations in life. They use a personal philosophy to guide them in their decision making, and in doing so, take active control of aspects of their care. Of course, if you choose not to be engaged in your medical care you will no doubt still find good treatment. In some ways, it can be easier to treat a patient who doesn't ask many questions. But if, like most patients, your goal is to navigate your cancer treatment, feeling as if you have control and options, you need to own some responsibility for it.

When someone says they have cancer, the first thing that comes to mind is that it seems complex. Cancer connotes mystery and difficulty. These words discourage you from understanding your illness. But it doesn't have to be so. I have long observed that while cancer is really many different diseases, dealing with its consequences requires a fundamental set of questions that all patients need to ask of their doctor and themselves

If you are feeling anxious, frightened, confused or simply don't know where to start, I hope to provide you comfort and practical advice through this book. I may not be seeing you in my office but I want to talk to you in the same way as I would a patient sitting before me. For almost everyone I have met, cancer is a difficult experience but not everything ends badly as you might fear. Modern medicine has the means to tackle disease like never before. Yes, we have a long way to go, but this is a really exciting time in oncology because of the marvellous gains we are making in our knowledge about how cancers behave. Knowledge of this behaviour translates into new drugs and other ways of treating cancer, and the changes are happening fast. I routinely use drugs that I had not heard of until just a few years ago. So while it's obviously a stretch to say you are lucky to have cancer now, you can take heart that doctors know more about your cancer now than they ever had earlier. The American Cancer Society estimates that someone diagnosed with cancer in the last decade has a five-year survival rate of 68 per cent compared to only a 49 per cent chance in the 1970s. However, there are serious outcomes that you may well need to prepare for. In saying this, I am not being pessimistic but honest, as you should expect me to be. Unfortunately, by not thinking of the right questions or not knowing how to ask them, you may never receive the answers that you need to plan ahead.

Reading this book will not make you a medical expert on your illness but I aspire to make you a more empowered patient. I hope to make you a patient who, no matter what the stage of your illness, feels prepared and knowledgeable, and is hence able to ask questions and make decisions wisely. Many people in your situation give up trying to understand their choices before they start because the road seems too hard. But I honestly believe that you will do yourself and your loved ones a favour by being informed.

So although your head may be spinning and there seems no end of things to think about, I urge you to sit down for a while and join me in making sense of what lies ahead. You are not alone.

1

What Is Cancer?

'Mrs Jordan?' I call out. A few seconds later, I raise my voice above the low din of the waiting room. 'Mrs Jordan, are you here?'

'Yes dear, I'm coming,' a bird-like voice emanates from behind a pillar. I crane my neck to follow the line of blue knitting yarn on the floor to its origin and find Mrs Jordan there. I join her to escort her into the consultation rooms and she huffs a little, covering the short distance to my room. Long-standing diabetes and heart disease have already taken a toll – she appears older than her stated seventy-six years. When she has sat down and caught her breath, I begin.

'Mrs Jordan, I am an oncologist. My role is to talk to you about your management after surgery. But first can you tell me a little bit about what you know?'

'All I know is that the surgeon got it all.'

'And did he tell you what it was?'

There is a knock on the door as a harried-looking woman walks in apologetically. She was trying to find a parking space. 'Sorry, this is my mum.'

Mrs Jordan smiles at her daughter, who takes her hand.

'I was telling the doctor that the surgeon took out the lump from my breast, dear.'

'What did he say it was?' I press.

'I don't know.'

'Mum, he told you the next day, remember?' her daughter prompts. 'Mum was very ill from the anaesthetic', she explains to me, 'and we were discharged soon after.'

'I don't remember being told anything else', Mrs Jordan says. 'Are you going to take my stitches out?'

'I am an oncologist. I treat cancer patients with chemotherapy and other drugs.'

'Oh, those poor people. Well, I just had a lump.'

Her daughter gently says, 'Mum, do you remember the surgeon telling you that the lump was cancerous?'

'No,' she frowns. 'I even saw the picture – it was a regular lump. Are you sure it was cancer?'

'You are right that the surgeon took it all out,' I tell her, 'but I am afraid it was breast cancer that he removed.'

We spend the next twenty minutes discussing the implications of having breast cancer and happily conclude that Mrs Jordan does not require chemotherapy, which relieves her no end.

'Blimey, I didn't even know I had cancer,' she says, scratching her chin as she departs.

Her daughter lingers in my room. 'Doctor, I'm sorry Mum is vague. You must think we are utter fools.'

I rush to reassure her that I experience variations of this conversation every day. Many patients are unsure of the terminology of cancer, which is not surprising as many health professionals use words like *tumour*, *lump*, *mass*, *spot*, *shadow* and *abnormality* as euphemisms. Does this sound familiar to you? On the other hand, you may hear the term *cancer* used repeatedly and still wonder exactly what it means. So much about cancer lends itself to misconception; so I want to spend some time explaining it in simple terms.

The word *cancer* comes from the Greek for *crab*, which a cancerous growth is thought to resemble. It is an uncontrolled growth of normal cells in any part of the body. Over time, the abnormal growth causes a lump (except in the case of blood cancers), although it may not necessarily be obvious to the touch. *Lump* is a generic word used to define many abnormalities, from a discrete mass to several little nodules and more. Cancer can arise in any part the body – from an organ like the bowel or brain to bone, cartilage or various types of blood cells.

Importantly, having a lump does not mean you have cancer. A biopsy can show whether a lump is benign or malignant. A *benign* lump is a growth that can cause irritating problems but generally doesn't threaten your life unless it occupies a particularly sensitive location, such as inside the skull or near a major blood vessel or nerve. A *malignant* lump is cancerous. It exhibits fast, abnormal growth, which can spread to distant parts of your body, and it has the capacity to cause damage and endanger life. However, I want to emphasize that not all cancers are equally aggressive, which is something we will discuss throughout the book.

Cancer is not one disease but actually hundreds of diseases that share some but not all characteristics. Since the diagnosis of cancer has such vast implications for you, it is important that you establish whether any lump, tumour or spot you have is cancerous. You need to understand this from the start, because I still meet patients who are stupefied to discover a cancer diagnosis even months into their treatment. 'But I thought they were treating a tumour,' a patient once protested in dismay when I casually asked her to remind me how long she had had cancer. I don't know who was more horrified – she, for discovering a clearer diagnosis, or me for blithely thinking that anyone receiving chemotherapy would surely associate it with cancer.

What causes cancer? As one patient recently said through a grimace: 'Everyone has a theory about what causes cancer. I just wish instead of inflicting it on me they would go and discover a cure. Now wouldn't that be useful?' Like many patients you may be questioning what might have led to the disease, puzzling over everything from smoking and diet to where you live and your stresses at work. This isn't helped by the fact that you will probably find many people who live pretty much similarly to you but who *don't* have cancer. While lung cancer is strongly associated with smoking, not all smokers get lung cancer. A healthy, lifelong vegetarian ends up with bowel cancer while his carnivorous, unfit brother doesn't. Your mother and daughter have breast cancer but you and your sister don't. Obviously this isn't a green light to live an unhealthy lifestyle (there are countless illnesses just as troublesome as cancer, and some worse), but it is a lesson that you are not in control of everything that goes astray in your body.

Put another way, cancer is not caused by a single factor you might easily determine, and is likely the result of many factors. Cancer also doesn't develop over days or weeks – it takes many months or years for the changes known as mutations to affect your cells and for cancer to become apparent. Patients are especially disappointed when they had been feeling well before their diagnosis. 'I ran a half-marathon two weekends ago, I can't possibly be sick,' one young patient insisted. But a closer look at his recent history revealed that he had been experiencing weight loss for the past three months and had put down his fatigue to athletic training. As commonly happens with pancreatic cancer, there was no clear warning sign until he became jaundiced over a period of two days. He then wondered whether there was something in his genes. It is certainly possible that he has a genetic predisposition to cancer (and we may not be able to find out), but it doesn't necessarily mean that his siblings are at increased risk of the same cancer. Scientists have defined genes that indicate a greater chance of developing cancer, but again, you may carry the gene and stay healthy. The majority of cancers are not related to inherited gene defects.

Age itself is a risk for getting cancer. Our cells replicate constantly during our lives. The more times they replicate, the greater the chances that an aberration will occur. However, the body is remarkable at self-correcting and it takes many aberrations for cancer to grow. Diet, smoking, exercise, stress, obesity, asbestos, pollution, radiation, geography, immune system changes, alcohol, infection and chemicals – all of these are linked to cancer but no one knows for sure in what way. Nobody can tell you definitely how much exposure to any of these might cause you to develop cancer or whether you ever will.

One of the more poignant things to confront at diagnosis is the guilt many patients feel for having developed cancer. You might find that you are blaming yourself or your loved one. Perhaps you are chastising yourself for not getting to the doctor earlier, for ignoring the nagging headache, for not having that blood test when it was due, or for wilfully avoiding paying attention to symptoms that you knew all along spelled trouble. You are not alone. In fact, you are just like most of us who want to stay as far away from doctors as possible and ignore things in the hope that they will go away. Often they do, but sometimes they don't. It is stressful and unhelpful to cast blame.

You should remind yourself that many factors have aligned to cause your cancer. Don't waste your time on what has gone before. Instead, join me in feeling optimistic about learning how to best navigate the way ahead.

Key Points

- Cancer is an abnormal, unregulated growth of cells that can occur in any part of the body.
- Cancer does not happen due to any one reason but a collection of genetic and environmental events.
- Not all cancers are the same, even if they sound similar in name or location. Don't automatically compare your cancer with that of other patients.
- Don't feel guilty about how or why cancer happened to you. Instead, arm yourself with the best ways of managing it.

2

Where Do I Even Begin?

I answer the phone one day to hear piercing sobs down the line and identify the voice to be that of an old friend, Allie, whom I haven't seen in some years. My heart beats heavily as I try to calm her, wondering what has gone wrong.

'You won't believe it, they say it's cancer,' she sobs. 'I have *cancer*. That's it, it's all over.'

I draw in my breath, jolted by the revelation

'I am going to die,' she declares heart-rendingly. 'I have never drunk, never smoked, exercised hard and eaten well. How can this happen to me?'

'Where is the cancer?' I ask after a while, unable to subdue the clinician in me as I listen to her anguish.

'What? Where is it? I had a mammogram and they detected this tiny little thing. I found out the results today, but there are other tests I need to have and I have no idea when they will operate because of the waiting lists. They think it's just in my breast but asked me to have other scans, which must mean they suspect it's everywhere. I know it's bad and that they're just not telling me. I mean, why else would they look so serious? And I have no idea whether to have the lump taken out, have a mastectomy, or even a double mastectomy so that I never have to go through this again. Part of me just wants to curl up and die now.'

My friend's anxiety and distress have allowed her imagination to run well ahead of the facts. Chances are that a mammogram-detected cancer is localized, operable and carries a very good prognosis. A localized breast cancer with no lymph node spread has a five-year survival rate of 99 per cent. The tests she is having are routine surveillance ones conducted in most patients. It is likely that the cancerous tumour will be removed without resorting to a mastectomy, let alone a bilateral (double) mastectomy, and she will lead a normal life again.

'I don't know who to tell,' she continues. 'Mum is nearly ninety and wouldn't take the news well. Patrick is overseas on an important business trip. Both the kids are interstate on exchange programmes. There is a lady at work who had breast cancer two years ago. She had a wretched time of it and I'm not sure if I want to know more. I was going to call my sister but she's so incredibly positive that she'd tell me to look on the bright side that it's *only* cancer. I just don't know ...'

'Allie, I am sorry about your diagnosis. It must have come as a complete shock.'

'I'm floored by this. I kept thinking that the biopsy was just a precautionary measure until the second the surgeon told me the result. I feel totally foolish because I have no idea what to do now. The surgeon told me a lot of things, gave me a pile of information, told me to have the tests, but now that I've walked out, I feel like I didn't hear any of it. But I can't bear to call back and ask anyone. What will they think of me?'

'Allie, where are you right now?'

'I've locked myself in my car. I'm too rattled to drive and I don't want to enter an empty house.'

'Stay put. I'll come and get you and we can go through these things together.'

Her relief is obvious. 'I don't expect you do that, but it would be just wonderful. Thank you.'

Allie and I drive to her house together. I am struck to see my usually in-control friend suddenly turned into a mass of uncertainty. She is not sure whether she wants to have tea or coffee, she calls her husband twice but hangs up before he answers, she paces the corridor, sits down and then gets up and starts pacing again. She asks me to tell her the best and worst of outcomes without sparing the details, but then decides she isn't really ready to hear either. She asks me how I can do my job and watch everyone dying all the time.

'But they don't die all the time, Allie,' I say, trying to reassure her.

'Of course they do. They have cancer,' she replies morosely.

I am filled with sympathy for her as I watch her transformation. I want to reassure her that she will be fine, but that would be premature and she would not forgive the false encouragement. I decide that what she really needs is help with the immediate practicalities. So I say, 'Allie, I'll help you in whatever way you want but let's start with a list of priorities.'

This strikes her normally practical self as a good idea. On a piece of paper, I write down in point form.

Book important scans and blood tests.

Call surgeon's office to ask about a second appointment or an operation date.

Inform Patrick, the kids and sister, Sarah.

On another piece of paper we decide on tasks to complete in the next few days.

Inform GP, discuss plans with her.

Tell Mum in person.

Call regular walking partner and next-door neighbour.

Tell immediate boss only. Hold off on telling other colleagues just yet.

By the third piece of paper, Allie feels up to writing the things she may want to do after surgery.

Find out about the oncologist a friend has praised. We agree that although I will be there for her, I should not be her primary doctor.

Locate useful patient literature on breast cancer.

Track down yoga teacher from years ago and re-enrol.

Tell wider circle of friends and colleagues.

Decide how much leave to take; consider the redundancy package offered last month.

Writing these lists takes just minutes but it has the immediate effect of making Allie regain a semblance of control. The task of dealing with the shock seems somewhat less daunting by breaking it into smaller elements, each of which seems possible to do in itself. Soon she feels her emotions have settled enough to call her husband, Patrick, and relay the news calmly. When he wants to cancel the rest of his trip she reassures him that she will be okay for the next few days and that she has made a list of priorities. She is also able to talk to her children in the same way. I notice that she keeps all her conversations short, enough to reassure her family that she is okay, but not long enough to become upset over the phone. 'There will be lots of time to talk over everything when we are together,' she tells them.

Despite my offer to stay, Allie decides to spend the night alone in her house, saying that at the end of a very emotional day she wants her own space. She says, frankly, 'I need to get my head around the diagnosis in a quiet space. This is a total shock but if I take some time to think things through, this will be good for us all.'

Over the next few days I watch Allie in admiration as she goes about her task. I once remark on the fact that she shares her news sparingly although she has no lack of caring people in her life. 'Do you not like talking about it?' I ask.

'A lot of advice is well intended but I find it confusing and maybe unnecessary. No one is short of an opinion on cancer but my immediate path is clear: I need to have an operation, so I want to keep a clear head and get through it.'

Allie's operation is followed by an uncomplicated recovery. It turns out that she has a small, low-grade tumour for which she is able to avoid chemotherapy. Prolonged medical leave is also not required and her accumulated annual leave covers her needs.

Some time later she reflects that many of her worst fears were never realized. 'But I would never have believed it at the time if you had told me. If I ever have to help somebody I must remember to just do useful things for them instead of trying to banish their fears.'

Fortunately, Allie is like many modern cancer patients who can expect to benefit from improving cure rates. Though the prevalence of cancer is high, the rate of death from cancer has gone down.

This success is more evident in the developed world. The World Health Organization (WHO) estimates that in 2012, cancer accounted for over eight million deaths. Many of these deaths occurred in low-income countries with scarce resources to diagnose and treat illness.

India faces a growing burden of cancer. One million cases are reported each year, with the figure set to double by 2025. The WHO estimates that there are over three million cancer patients in India with up to 700,000 dying of the disease each year.

India has a somewhat unique pattern of cancer compared to other countries. Cancers of the lung and oral cavity, lip, throat and neck are the most common among men, resulting from cigarette and oral tobacco consumption. Women suffer more from cervical, breast and ovarian cancers. India leads the world in cancers of the oral cavity, gall bladder and cervix. A particular problem is very late diagnosis, which means that the majority of patients, 70 per cent, die in their first year. And unlike developed countries, many more deaths occur in youth and in the productive years of life.

Doctors say the causes of such a high incidence of cancer relate to internal factors like genes, hormones and poor immune conditions, and external or environmental factors like food habits, industrialization, overgrowth of population and lifestyle. Lack of public awareness, insufficient medical facilities, poor ratio of doctors to patients and delayed diagnosis all contribute to cancer being a feared 'killer' disease although, if detected in its early stages, cancer can be effectively treated. Health illiteracy and the stigma associated with the disease coupled with the shortage of cancer specialists means that nearly 80 per cent of cancer patients seek help too late and that too from health providers who are not familiar with cancer.

Nevertheless, as the world becomes a global village, Indian cancer patients are benefiting from new developments. One of modern oncology's miracles is Herceptin, an antibody used against certain forms of breast cancer. When I was a trainee oncologist the drug was just coming into use in clinical trials. What we could tell women was that the limited global experience with Herceptin looked positive. A short time later, results started arriving, confirming that the addition of Herceptin to routine chemotherapy improved survival. They were heady times – encouraged by the positive results I remember combing through medical records to recall women to clinic who were eligible for Herceptin. The use of Herceptin is now so common that the memory seems almost quaint. Today's oncology trainee does not know a time that Herceptin was not available. And by the time that trainee concludes her training, you can be assured that she will be using drugs she has yet to hear of.

The way Allie dealt with the blow of her diagnosis is instructive. You can assume that it is common to follow very little of the initial conversation about a cancer diagnosis. Often, everything becomes just a hum after the first time you hear that you have cancer. It is helpful to request written information as well as a copy of any results. You or someone in your family may feel like reading it at some stage. Have someone jot some notes in the doctor's room about the kind of cancer it is, if it has spread and how it is to be treated. Find out whom you can call with other questions – usually a doctor or a chemotherapy nurse. Some doctors might be comfortable with you recording their consultation so that you might want to ask.

When you emerge with a new diagnosis of cancer your mind will be in a spin. You will probably feel emotional, lost and unsure what the next step is. This is entirely normal. Many patients describe feeling like an automaton in the next days and weeks. They go through the motions hoping that one day things will make sense.

The good news is that things do begin to fall into place as you learn the new language of dealing with cancer. It is an entirely new experience. You will meet medical professionals who seem very knowledgeable and completely at ease with a diagnosis that has overturned your world. Sometimes you may not understand their language and wonder whether they have any grasp of the turmoil in your life, but know that they care deeply for you and will always be looking for better ways to treat you. You will also come across patients in the waiting room, in support groups and in adjoining chemotherapy chairs – hard as it is to believe, some of them will become your friends. Some people look very sick and some so well that you wonder what they are doing there. Don't compare yourself to any other patient – you don't know what their precise experience is, even if they tell you they have the same cancer.

Be easy on yourself. Allow for tears and moments of bewilderment or desperation. But also let some hope through by telling yourself that at this very new stage of your disease nobody possesses all the answers. More and more cancers have effective treatments that were hardly imaginable a decade ago. With modern communication it is very easy for doctors to exchange information and advice about even rare diseases. And there is constant new research to inform management. Of course, there is no opportune time to have cancer, but when I look back at the ten years during which I have been an oncologist, I recognize how much more sophisticated we have become at treating cancer and its consequences in that time.

You have control over your response to a new diagnosis of cancer. Everyone feels completely helpless at some time but you can acknowledge this, make allowances for it and still feel optimistic that after the initial shock you will proactively try to regain some control.

Perhaps you too can begin by constructing a few lists that cover tasks from the very important to the desirable. Pace yourself. Surround yourself with support but be discerning. For example, you may not appreciate someone repeatedly telling you that you will be fine when they don't know the full story. Or you may not want to hear someone else's pessimistic or far-fetched tales about someone they know who had cancer. There are people who will tell you to cry 'to let it all out' and others who will forbid you from ever feeling weak. Of course, none of this advice is absolutely right or wrong. What is useful is to choose one or two people who can offer quiet, respectful support and a ready ear but who are not dogmatic about how you should respond to your situation, because this is something that only you can determine. You are the person driving your management. The value in this will become more apparent as we move into the next few chapters to do with practical elements of cancer treatment.

Key Points

- Expect many things to be a blur when you are first diagnosed with cancer.
- Seek the help of those who quietly and respectfully support you without rushing you into decisions.
- Write down your immediate tasks – dismantling a large problem into small elements makes it easier to tackle.
- You are the patient and you should be in control – it's okay to take some time to get there.

3

How Is Cancer Treated?

It was one of my earliest chemotherapy prescriptions. 'Here you are,' I said, handing a pile of paperwork to the patient. 'Give this to the nurses, they will organize everything. And call me if you have any questions.'

The patient hesitated. 'Actually doctor, I do have a question right now.'

'Yes?'

'I know I'm having chemo, but … what is it?'

I am sure she noticed my crestfallen expression. I had just spent thirty minutes discussing chemotherapy with her and she apparently had no idea what I had been talking about. Surely I hadn't been so poor in my explanation, yet one look at her face confirmed that she had been nodding along to my words without understanding.

'Which bit don't you understand?'

'Well, what *is* chemo? Is there an operation involved? I know there are injections, so is it sort of like having a flu shot? What I really don't understand is, how does the chemo know where to go in my body?'

The patient warmed up as she saw me listening intently. 'I apologize, doctor, but I'm only just beginning to get my head around this stuff. I'm fifty years old and consider myself reasonably well informed but I can tell you that this is all completely new and unsettling.'

I was touched by her honesty. 'That's fine. Tell me first, what other questions can you think of?'

'Like everyone else, I've heard that chemo is awful but someone said that radiation is better, and others say I should try non-traditional medicine or having a one-off operation to remove all the bad seeds. This is all like learning a new language. So I know I am taking up your time, but if you can explain to me in the simplest language possible how cancer is treated and what these options actually mean, I'd be really grateful.'

It was a reminder that what was normal, everyday practice for me as a doctor was a confronting experience for her. I realized how easily I had slipped into medical jargon. So I set about answering her questions using more plain language. I was wary of oversimplifying things, but her request had been clear. What is the nature of the problem, what kinds of treatments are available, what is the general thrust of their different approaches, and why might doctors recommend one or the other at different times?

At the end of our consultation, I was rewarded with a grateful smile. She said, 'Not only is this really the first time that I understand things, but I daresay I will feel more confident explaining it to others.'

If you have been recently diagnosed with cancer, I am sure your mind is swirling with thoughts, suggestions and recommendations. These days everybody has a cancer story to share and many patients complain that they feel even more confused after talking with others. But in order to make sense of the choices being presented you need to understand a little of the basic terminology of cancer treatment, so let me take you through it in easy-to-understand terms.

The study, diagnosis and treatment of cancer constitute the branch of medicine known as oncology. The medical professionals you will likely deal with, apart from your local GP, family physician or internist, are oncologists (my profession), surgeons and radiotherapists. Common ways of treating cancer include surgery (an operation to remove affected areas), chemotherapy (often simply referred to as *chemo*), radiotherapy (or *radiation*), hormonal therapy and targeted therapy (also known as biological therapy). These are sometimes prescribed in combination, or one as a preparation for the other, or as an alternative when one treatment has not achieved the desired result.

Chemotherapy refers to drugs that kill rapidly dividing cancer cells by disrupting their life cycle. The drugs are administered through the bloodstream, so they affect the person's whole body in order to be sure they treat the cancer. Chemotherapy is not one drug, but a tailored combination of numerous drugs that can be given through injection into the veins (intravenously); injection into the muscle, an artery, the abdominal cavity, into an organ, under the skin; or as a pill or skin cream. The method mostly depends on the type and location of the cancer. Most commonly, chemotherapy is given intravenously, usually in your arm. In some patients, a thin and flexible plastic tube called a port may be inserted into a larger vein in the arm or neck and left on a long-term basis, so that ongoing chemotherapy can be simply hooked up to the tube. Port insertion is a minor surgical procedure that takes place under local anaesthetic or light sedation. It allows nurses to take blood samples and deliver chemotherapy easily without any difficulty locating an appropriate vein each time.

People receive chemotherapy for different reasons. It may be to cure cancer, to stabilize or slow cancer growth, or to provide relief from troublesome symptoms from a tumour, such as pain or pressure. Depending on the disease, chemotherapy can be given prior to an operation (pre-operative or *neo-adjuvant* treatment), after an operation (post-operative or *adjuvant* treatment), or without being associated with an operation. It can be combined with radiotherapy or one of the other therapies mentioned above if it makes your treatment more effective overall. Chemotherapy doses are calculated based on your height, weight and other characteristics, such as organ function and overall well-being. Depending on the nature of the cancer being treated, it is administered on different schedules, which might be daily, weekly or monthly. The drugs in chemotherapy are toxic and, as they are administered to the whole body through the blood, they affect healthy cells as well as cancerous ones. So chemotherapy has a range of side effects, usually manageable with attentive care. Most patients with cancer end up receiving some form of chemotherapy, which tends to continue for a long time. So you will find me returning to discuss the nuances of chemotherapy in future chapters.

Radiotherapy for cancer commonly involves a machine that directs high-energy radiation to kill cancer cells (*external beam radiotherapy*). Unlike chemotherapy, radiotherapy's effects are confined to the area exposed to it. Other radiotherapy methods you may come across include the injection of a radioactive substance into your veins (*systemic radiotherapy*) or the placement of a radioactive seed (*brachytherapy*) into the part of the body affected by cancer. Radiotherapy techniques are continually being improved with the common aim of targeting the tumour but sparing normal tissue and limiting the treatment time. You may hear terms like *intensity-modulated radiotherapy*, *radiosurgery*, *gamma knife* and others during your treatment. These are specialized techniques that your radiation oncologist will explain further if they apply to you.

Many patients will receive radiotherapy somewhere along the line during their cancer treatment, but it is unusual to have it as the sole treatment unless you are not fit to receive chemotherapy. If you have metastatic, or in other words, advanced cancer, you may receive radiotherapy to a problematic part of the cancer but rely on chemotherapy to address the rest of the disease. Whole-body radiotherapy is very toxic and not used in the treatment of organ cancers although it is in some forms of blood cancers. Radiotherapy may be combined with chemotherapy to cure a tumour or shrink it to enable an operation. It may be used after surgery to kill cells that are thought to remain and, like chemotherapy, it can also be used against a tumour causing pain, pressure or other irritating symptoms. Your radiotherapy dose is calculated by the radiation oncologist with the help of computer simulation. Detailed scans show the exact location of the tumour and its relationship to surrounding tissue, helping to direct the radiotherapy to the right site. When you are receiving radiotherapy it is important for patients to maintain the same position every day, so your skin may be marked with small tattoos and you may be asked to wear a special mask or other device. Like chemotherapy, the duration of radiotherapy varies depending on what is being treated and with what goal. For example, treatment intended to cure the cancer may be more prolonged than that meant to ease symptoms (*palliative radiotherapy*). Despite the care that is taken to target radiotherapy exactly, it also affects normal surrounding tissue, leading to side effects. Side effects of radiotherapy depend on the area being treated – they include nausea, dry skin, local pain and skin breakdown, infection, diarrhoea, incontinence, reduced fertility, and memory and attention problems. Second cancers can occur at sites treated with radiotherapy although this usually requires a lag period of decades. Some areas of the body are more sensitive to radiation than others and it is sometimes not possible to treat an area again if cancer returns to it because the treatment may do more harm than good. Side effects can be short and long term and many can be managed with meticulous attention throughout treatment.

Hormonal therapy refers to the use of hormones to curb cancer. They can be given in tablet or injectable form and have long been used to treat diseases that rely on hormonal influence to grow, such as breast, prostate and gynaecological cancers. Treatment is given to block or otherwise manipulate this influence. While the side effects of hormonal therapy are usually not as severe as those of chemotherapy and radiotherapy, hormonal treatment is not without its set of consequences. For example, testosterone and estrogen are the chief male and female sex hormone respectively. Their deprivation can cause a list of problems including fatigue, hot flushes, osteoporosis, arthritis, weight gain, sexual and cognitive dysfunction. Not everyone will experience all these problems; some people will have a fairly smooth experience on them and many will either become accustomed to minor issues or find ways of overcoming them. On the other hand, some patients develop unacceptable toxicity and must come off hormonal therapy.

Targeted or biological therapy is a fast-moving, new area of oncology. Again, taken as pills or injection, targeted therapy hones in on the precise biological mechanism by which cancer cells are thought to grow, altering them in some way to kill them or prevent them spreading. This is a more personalized form of therapy than chemotherapy, which is now sometimes described as a blunt instrument against cancer. Targeted therapy (or biological therapy) might block a particular protein related to cell growth, cancer spread or blood vessel development, or it might stimulate the body's own immune system to attack cancer.

Targeted therapy is the holy grail of cancer medicine. With it, doctors hope to deliver treatment to the exact site it is needed without upsetting surrounding healthy tissues. The more precisely we know why your cancer developed, the better we might be able to treat it by targeting the biological pathways that have gone astray. This is called personalized therapy and is a very active and exciting area of research. Oncologists and researchers are still learning to use targeted therapies properly. Many are being widely used, and when a targeted therapy seems to be effective in one cancer, researchers are keen to study its effect on another cancer. The curious thing is that a drug that yields good results on one type of cancer is not always effective at treating another cancer, which demonstrates that all cancers are different.

The side effects of biological therapy are still being finessed. Broadly speaking they tend to be less toxic than chemotherapy or radiotherapy and thus they should preserve your quality of life. However, even these therapies cannot fully isolate their target, which means that surrounding normal tissues are affected contributing to toxicity. The side effects are severe in some cases but the advent of targeted therapies has allowed many patients to lead a better quality of life with limited or manageable side toxicity. It is worth knowing that a lot of these therapies still need to be combined with chemotherapy. Oncologists call this using a chemotherapy backbone, which means that although your targeted therapy itself is not toxic, the added chemotherapy may produce or exacerbate toxicity.

Chemotherapy, hormonal therapy and targeted therapies might be taken at home or administered in an outpatient clinic or a hospital inpatient ward, depending on your needs. Radiotherapy requires specialized machines, necessitating your travel to a centre as an outpatient, usually back and forth every day for the duration of the treatment. If you are very unwell or need urgent radiotherapy you may be admitted to a hospital as an inpatient.

One thing you may notice is how often the phrase 'depending on your cancer' is used. This is not an attempt to avoid a deeper discussion of your options. I guarantee that there will be plenty of opportunities for that. But if there is one thing I would like you to take away from this chapter, it is this: Think of cancer treatment, and specifically chemotherapy, as a wide canopy. How and whether it cures you, protects you from recurrence or relieves your symptoms is determined by a number of things. These include your age and coexisting ailments (especially those that affect major organs such as your heart, kidneys, lungs and liver), the type of cancer you have, where it is, if it has spread and what the goals of care are. Unfortunately, the goal of care is not always cure because of the stage of the cancer. And, of course, it is also dependent on your own philosophy about what you are prepared to accept and whether you agree with the statistical definition or your doctor's definition of benefit. We will explore these issues in later chapters.

This brings me to a quick mention of stage. Amongst the top five questions patients and carers ask is, 'What stage is the cancer at?' If I can break down the understanding of almost everyone who asks this question, it is that stage four is bad and the rest they are not so sure about. Many people also know that spread to the bones or liver denotes stage four disease, but they don't know what the other three stages really mean. 'All I know is that it's not the final stage, so I am safe', one patient said, only to be disappointed when she found out that she wasn't out of the woods with a lower stage of cancer whose pathology was aggressive.

Stage describes the extent and severity of cancer. It is a short form of describing where the cancer has spread and allows oncologists to talk to each other in a common language and do things like read and understand the literature, plan treatment, and assess whether a clinical trial is appropriate for you.

The commonest form of staging is based on the TNM system. T stands for tumour size, N for the number of lymph nodes involved, M for the presence and location of metastases. Based on a clinical exam, surgery, pathology, X-rays or other relevant facts your cancer is assigned a stage. The definitions of stage can change periodically and more than one type of tumour spread can fit into a stage. So many oncologists prefer to define the T, N and M. For example, a Stage III cancer can be a large tumour (T3) with no nodes (N0) or metastases (M0) or a slightly smaller tumour (T2) with lymph nodes involved (N2) and no distant metastases (M0). However, we know that lymphatic involvement in cancer poses an additional risk. Similarly, while metastases are important, it is equally important to know where they are located. Involvement of the liver is usually more critical than the bones. Tiny lung metastases may not cause any problem but cancerous fluid in the lung can seriously impact breathing. It is important to note that tumours also don't affect you in a predictable way from one stage to the other. Some people with widely metastatic disease feel better than their counterparts with less disease burden.

My advice to patients is that rather than asking about the stage of the cancer, a nebulous concept for many, find out how your body is involved with the disease. Ask where the primary cancer is, whether the lymph nodes are involved and what other organs are affected. Ask how aggressive the cancer seems and what the likely future course is. This detailed information is a far better basis for you to explore your options.

When exploring options, one of the commonest reasons for consternation amongst cancer patients is when they compare their treatment to that someone else is having. 'My friend's father has lung cancer and he is on a totally different pill than me.' 'When my sister got breast cancer, the surgeon operated on it straight away. Why must I have chemo?' 'A lady at work had no side effects at all from a new radiotherapy machine but I can't get out of bed. What have they done to me?' Other comparisons involve dosing, schedule, frequency of tests and other details. 'How can one pill be the same as four hours of chemo? Are you sure I will be okay?' 'My mum had the exact same cancer and needed one month of radiotherapy, but they stopped my dad's treatment after a few days. That doesn't make sense.' 'My friend sees a specialist who does scans every six months but I don't get that. Should I be worried?'

These are all good questions because they represent patient engagement. You should understand fundamental aspects of your treatment and be an advocate for yourself. But beware of superficial comparisons because every cancer truly is different and every patient requires and deserves individual attention, drug modification and monitoring. Even if you start out on the same treatment as the person sitting next to you in the chemotherapy unit, a small reduction in your dose may prove beneficial due to the reduction in toxicity, while stopping her chemotherapy completely before yours is finished might confer equivalent benefit.

So I hope you see that you are reliant on your doctors to tailor your prescription to your needs, which is why it is important to find somebody whom you can talk to and who will heed your goals of care. We will go into lot more details as I share other helpful tips with you to make your journey easier.

Key Points

- Cancer connotes many different diseases – it is not helpful to compare treatments with other patients.
- Look at cancer therapy as a wide canopy. Whether it cures you completely, slows down progression or relieves troublesome symptoms depends on a number of factors that your oncologist will explain. Your cancer may need more than one form of therapy.
- The precise treatment you receive will be tailored to your circumstances and what your body will tolerate.
- Rather than asking what stage of cancer you have, try to understand what organs are involved, how you are affected and how treatment will make a difference. This is a far more practical consideration that will help you assess the benefit of treatment.

4

Finding an Oncologist

We receive news of cancer harder than perhaps any other diagnosis, despite there being other illnesses, diseases and conditions with more grim prospects of recovery. Being diagnosed with cancer is frightening and upsetting in an especially acute way, worse than end-stage renal failure, emphysema or even severe heart failure, or the many neurological disorders that lend themselves to a poor quality and limited extent of life. Perhaps this is because some diseases are less visible due to their lower prevalence while others simply don't strike people as being life-threatening in the same way as cancer, which in its advanced stages causes a visible and inexorable decline.

As a patient put it to me: 'When I heard I had cancer, my first thought was that I was dying. Eight years later, I am fit and well, but my cousin, who had a major stroke around the same time, died just one year after diagnosis. I remember thinking they had lots of cures for his problem of blood pressure and I would be the one who would die first. It only sank in later that despite having the label "cancer" attached to me, my diagnosis was far more favourable than my poor cousin's.'

The language of cancer is couched in uncertainty. When there is so much emotion and fear associated with a diagnosis, it is difficult to separate emotion from facts. This makes it harder for patients to ask the right questions and understand information, and difficult for the oncologist to cover everything that the patient might desire.

It is likely that if you have cancer you will eventually meet an oncologist, a specialist doctor trained in the management of cancers. The exception is patients with very early-stage cancer that has been completely removed by a surgeon who is confident no other treatment is required. As increasing numbers of cancer cases are being discovered early through screening, this situation is becoming more common. But the majority of cancer patients will need an oncologist.

An oncologist typically prescribes chemotherapy and manages other aspects of cancer. While you may have other kinds of treatment, chemotherapy is the most common treatment for a variety of cancers. Oncologists who deal with childhood cancers are known as paediatric oncologists. You may also come across the term radiation oncologist, which describes a different type of specialist, one who treats cancer with radiation therapy as opposed to chemotherapy. Not every patient with cancer requires radiotherapy, or chemotherapy for that matter. If your cancer needs radiotherapy it is most likely that either a surgeon or an oncologist will refer you to a radiation oncologist, but don't be anxious if you never meet one.

Long-term management of cancer typically includes chemotherapy and dealing with an oncologist; so finding someone you like is important. You may not realize it now but your relationship with your oncologist will become one of the most significant in your life. If you are receiving chemotherapy you will spend more time with your oncologist than many family members. When you finish chemotherapy you will regularly return to your oncologist and rely on him or her to guide you through the next phase of your treatment, whatever that may be. You will want your oncologist to not only explain complicated medical information but also to put it in perspective so that you can understand what's important to you. A patient who sought a second opinion from me said, 'The first oncologist said, "Don't worry about it, it's nothing serious." Of course I want to believe him but he sounded so casual that I don't know if I can.' What he was saying is that he wanted to know he could trust his doctor.

Naturally, you want to know that if things change, your oncologist will be on the front foot and is fully aware of your condition and history. Most importantly, you want to feel comfortable opening up to him or her. The relationship might well last many years, so finding the right oncologist for you is important.

What does an oncologist do? Once, before the routine use of chemotherapy began in the late 1970s, oncologists had limited options in how they could help a suffering patient. What they mostly offered were sympathy and consolation, while expressing private frustration at their inability to tackle the root cause. Modern oncology, though, has delivered doctors with an embarrassment of riches in terms of medical treatments that they can employ for different patients, and a continual stock of innovations. In short, then, an oncologist is largely a chemotherapy doctor, but I would like to think that we do much more than that.

Let me tell you about my role as an oncologist. My patients' primary expectation is that I know how to treat their cancer. But they also expect that I will be a trusted partner with whom they can discuss thorny issues that arise during a cancer diagnosis, whether they relate to workplace troubles, tension with an unsupportive spouse, or questions about whether the toxicities of treatment are worth it for them. On different days they expect me to vary my tone and concern for them, recognizing when they are fragile and need me to skirt carefully around emotional subjects, or when they need clear, unequivocal advice.

You can imagine why many patients experience the lack of a meaningful engagement with their oncologist. Sometimes it is not possible for one doctor to be all things; other times, an oncologist is not prepared or able to meet all the patient's needs. Some oncologists feel most comfortable managing chemotherapy and leaving other elements of care to a variety of professionals better suited to the task. Others take a more inclusive approach. I don't think there is anything necessarily right or wrong with either. Certainly, some patients feel that they would rather have their oncologist concentrate on medical matters and leave things like psychological support, nutritional advice and discussion of welfare benefits to others. Others want their oncologist to help them in broader ways. Take some time to think about your preferences and appreciate the nuances of different oncologists. Ask around for recommendations. This way, you can save yourself unnecessary frustration or disappointment.

A patient in her eighties put it to me like this: 'Every doctor I see wants to look at the computer, fill out the script, write the notes, take my pulse and measure the lump all at the same time. Then there are a dozen questions fired at me followed by directions. Where is the time to talk?' This spirited woman was identifying a common sentiment amongst patients that they need time and simplified explanations to truly understand their choices. In her frustration she changed oncologists and was satisfied with the outcome, but of course, most patients don't do that. They suffer their dissatisfaction silently, but the effects are enduring, not only on the patient but also the family.

Over the years I have heard patients report a number of reasons for their dissatisfaction with my colleagues and me. For some, the lack of information rankles. 'For all the time I have spent in the chemotherapy chair, I can't say I really understand what's going on,' a young woman mused. For others, information is plentiful but doesn't make sense. 'I don't care about the blood count or the numbers – they don't mean anything', a burly farmer grumbled. 'I just know that I feel terrible but no one seems to listen.' Many feel rushed for time with the oncologist or find that the atmosphere of the consultation does not allow them to voice their true feelings. A colleague of mine used to accompany his late father to an oncologist. 'The doctor's facial expression was never one to invite questions. My dad would never dare to ask him anything if it weren't for me nudging him along, and even I felt reluctant. I found the oncologist quite unreceptive to our need for information.'

And yet, on a recent ward round, I was gratified to hear a patient say of her oncologist: 'He is a gift from heaven as far as I am concerned. No matter how busy he is, he has time for my questions. He always drops in when I am having chemotherapy, and if he is running late he tells the nurses. I've been seeing him for two years and sometimes I doubt I would have lived as long had it not been for his kindness and care.' I know her oncologist – and his extraordinarily busy schedule – well, but the patient was so genuinely appreciative of his help that I found myself reflecting again and again on the skills that he has honed in order to serve his patients so well.

The sister of an intellectually disabled cancer patient told me that her brother benefited greatly from the caring nature of his oncologist. 'She always speaks softly to him and doesn't make sudden movements, which frighten him. He is wary of doctors but she is the only one he will allow near him. Her ability to spot his discomfort is very reassuring to us.'

Nowhere is the doctor–patient relationship more deeply impacting, with the potential to have an enduring effect, than in oncology. Within a short span of time, at an emotionally intense period in their lives, cancer patients end up spending a lot of hours with their oncologist. Therefore, it is only natural to expect this relationship to be one of mutual comfort and respect. So let's discuss how you might find an oncologist suited to your needs. On a checklist for finding an oncologist, what are the essentials and what are the desirables?

The first concern for many patients is whether their oncologist is adequately trained. In India, the answer is yes, with the qualification that there are still too few training positions relative to the population in need. A primary medical degree must be recognized by the Medical Council of India and be followed by an MD (Doctor of Medicine) in internal medicine. The requirements to enter an oncology fellowship programme are robust. Desirable qualities for these competitive posts include having prior experience in a structured training programme, exposure to a large academic centre, an interest in clinical research and a commitment to interpersonal communication.

Like many other countries, an oncology fellowship in India lasts two years, with many doctors motivated to extend their training and build their expertise in a particular area by training or working abroad. These days, major international societies actively encourage and sponsor doctors from developing countries to gain international exposure. In the era of Internet-based communication, there has generally been an increasing flow of medical knowledge and expert advice, which has particularly benefited patients in underserved areas, in India and elsewhere.

A qualified oncologist has a few choices available with respect to workplace. He or she may find a position in an academic hospital, which provides access to research, training and mentoring. A large private hospital system with better facilities and access to a range of interventions might suit others. Some doctors may work both in the public and the private system.

Where an oncologist practises is not necessarily the best indication of his or her qualities because the venue of work depends on many personal and professional factors. Some oncologists prefer the academic setting of a large public hospital where there is room for collegial collaboration, teaching and mentoring, and access to expansive research facilities. Patient care and on-call duties are shared amongst oncologists on a rostered basis at a public hospital, which often suits parents of young children, for example. Others find they are better suited to working independently and having more direct control over their patients' care. Private practice is financially more rewarding but it comes with an entirely different set of demands, including the capacity to manage a practice and employees, stringent after-hours commitments and the lack of the public hospital infrastructure and support systems. Both systems have their benefits and drawbacks.

From the patient's viewpoint, it is important to understand some facts. Anyone who is a qualified medical oncologist possesses the same basic set of skills, with standards that are very high and routinely reviewed. Modern cancer treatment has a good evidence base and consists of a large number of standardized treatment regimens, which means that your cancer should be treated in roughly the same way regardless of where you live. The place where an oncologist works or the number of degrees your oncologist has is not a good measure of how you will relate to your doctor.

The decision to undergo treatment in a public or private hospital is obviously made for you if you don't have private health insurance. I reassure my Australian patients that they will receive a high standard of care in the public hospital system, which draws on a large pool of talent. Depending on the country and the sophistication of the medical system, there can be discrepancies in access and applying the standard of care. In India, private health care is not readily available everywhere. Even where it is available, it is not affordable for everyone.

An important practical distinction between private and public hospital treatment of cancer relates to the patient's relationship with an oncologist. If you see an oncologist in private practice, you enter into a contract with that individual, who will then guide you through treatment. In many, but not all, public health care networks, your contract is with a few oncologists. Some hospitals have a policy of assigning a patient to a particular oncologist as frequently as possible while others don't, and patient care is shared amongst what is usually a small and long-term team of specialists. Your first reaction on reading this may be that it will be quite dislocating to have a number of doctors involved in your care. While the majority of patients cope quite well and even appreciate the advantage of obtaining a different viewpoint, some patients could do with a more regular and firmer relationship with one oncologist. It may help you to know that over the course of their illness, it is not unusual for patients to utilize both the public and private hospital systems, dictated in part by the type of insurance they have and in part by the unique resources available in a large public hospital. The bottom line is that if you don't have the option of private insurance, don't stress, because luckily, it is not fundamental to your care.

When you hear that you have cancer, there is an acute and understandable anxiety to source the best person at the best centre for your treatment. This makes patients flock to places whose name they hear most frequently. Finding a quality centre is important, but remember that just because a public or private hospital is said to be the best doesn't mean that it will serve your individual interests well. A bustling academic hospital can still let you down by failing to monitor your side effects closely, while the smaller hospital around the corner, with fewer doctors, may just have the time to discuss those same effects at greater length and pull you back from the brink of disaster. Seeing a private oncologist may be costly but for you the continuity of care might make it worth it. On the other hand, you might find that attending a public hospital outpatients department with its mix of different oncologists serves you better. Sometimes, especially if you have an uncommon cancer, what you need most is the combination of medical expertise, experience and technology that only a top academic centre can muster. Just like your health, your needs are dynamic and the best oncologist is one who can stay in tune with them.

Patients often fret over whether they are seeing the right expert for their condition. One of the commonest questions I am asked by acquaintances is whether somebody they are seeing is an expert in their particular kind of cancer, such as breast, pancreatic or lung cancer. I see people bypassing their local facilities to travel at great effort and cost to consult somebody recommended as the best doctor for their cancer. Since cancer care is a long-term undertaking, the logistics that don't seem much in the beginning soon become onerous, and in many cases, of questionable worth. There are definitely instances, such as the diagnosis of an uncommon or rare cancer, where highly experimental treatment needs rigorous monitoring, or where such care has been specifically recommended by doctors, that it is important to seek out especially expert advice. But for cancers most common in the population, such as breast, lung, gastrointestinal or prostate, many oncologists treat these competently.

Due to the explosion in treatments for many cancers, it is becoming increasingly true that oncologists themselves define or limit the types of cancers they treat, but this rarely means that an oncologist who advertises his practice as being predominantly that of lung cancer cannot treat your prostate cancer well, provided he accepts you as a patient. By accepting you as a patient the oncologist is declaring in good faith that he or she can manage your cancer. For those specialists who only see patients with a certain type of cancer – this seems especially true of the commonest cancers – it is naturally true that the greater volume of these cancers they see may provide them with a more nuanced experience that can sometimes be useful. But countries like the United Kingdom, Canada and Australia do not have the same numbers of cancer patients as a country like the United States (1.5 million new cases per year), which can sustain entire careers or centres dedicated to the treatment of one particular cancer. In smaller places an oncologist is more likely to specialize in more than one tumour 'stream', as it is known. In large countries like India, there aren't enough oncologists and therefore, doctors must treat more than one type of cancer to meet patients' needs.

The bottom line is that for a common cancer there are standard guidelines for treatment that can be safely applied by an oncologist. If your oncologist does require expert advice, it is easily available over the phone, Internet, and by direct consultation. Hence the need to find the right expert should be tempered by an understanding of the relative value of this endeavour for you.

So if all qualified oncologists have a basic skill set that is of a high level, if private or public hospital care doesn't necessarily matter to every patient, and locating an expert among experts is not essential for many cancer patients, what should determine the choice of an oncologist? In my opinion it is the ability to communicate. While medical knowledge is freely available, it is the ability to explain it to a patient in an accessible way and to do so with empathy, patience and sensitivity that sets apart a good oncologist.

You may be thinking that finding such an oncologist would simply be a matter of luck but there is more to it. Oncologists genuinely care about their patients – otherwise they would not choose to work in a field so rich with human suffering. But like other people, oncologists may express their caring for you in different ways. For some, it means passionate laboratory-based research or launching aggressive attempts at cure, for others it means paying equal attention to your emotional health. Some oncologists are always serious and businesslike while others like to inject the occasion with some levity. Some oncologists spend longer on an appointment than others.

The first step towards finding an oncologist is figuring out what you want. You may be someone who just wants the facts and don't expect or need an oncologist to hold your hand. You might thrive on facts and statistics, studying them to determine your next step, or you might put more faith in your oncologist's judgement and leave it to him or her to make the critical decisions. Ask yourself how you deal with uncertainty. If your oncologist demonstrated uncertainty about treatment options, would you lose confidence because she didn't have a ready answer or would you be reassured that she was candidly reflecting the availability of a range of options and not pretending to be certain which is best? In my experience, patients want a little bit of all of the above. They want a doctor whose competence is beyond reproach because, after all, the primary goal of coming to an oncologist is receiving good treatment. But then they want someone sympathetic, someone who will listen and respond accordingly, and walk in step with them. Prominent themes in cancer include doubt, vulnerability, and the fear of abandonment. Cancer patients want to be treated by someone who will infuse their life with hope and accompany them on the whole journey, not just the phase of active chemotherapy. In other words, they want an oncologist who will appreciate that the art of oncology is as important as its science.

The usual ways of meeting an oncologist are through a surgeon who has operated on your cancer, through a reference from your GP or through a private or public hospital where you have been admitted for an illness that turns out to be cancer-related. In almost all these circumstances your referring doctor has a professional relationship with the oncologist. A breast surgeon typically sends her patients to one or two oncologists; a cardiothoracic surgeon works alongside a few lung cancer experts; a urologist has links with certain prostate cancer specialists and so on. Surgeons and oncologists may share the same offices, with a tacit agreement to refer patients to each other. A GP usually has a list of medical oncologists in the local area, some of whom may have introduced themselves in person when they began practice. With a typical GP having a small handful of cancer patients under his care, he would get to know their oncologists via correspondence and conversations. He may have had to call an oncologist for urgent advice and may have been impressed, or dissatisfied, by the speed or the content of the advice. Like so many other instances in life, these impressions play a role in the decision to refer a new patient to an oncologist. In a public hospital, there is usually a roster of oncologists who provide consultations and then direct patients to the most appropriate clinic for treatment. Depending on the day, you might see someone different. Depending on the system that hospital employs, you may see the same oncologist again for later visits or be cared for by a team of doctors. If there is a team-care arrangement, there will be some constant elements, such as certain senior doctors and nurses, alongside a changing roster of trainees on placement, medical students and the like. Your treatment will still be determined by an oncologist.

If you have the time, one way to find a suitable oncologist is to ask other people, perhaps cancer patients, your GP, a specialist, a cancer support group or other medical and nursing staff involved in your care. Ask them what they like about the oncologist they recommend. Ask what he would charge. Are his patients satisfied with his care? Does he encourage questions? Is he willing to listen to your point of view or strict about his advice? Does he keep your GP abreast of important changes to your management?

Occasionally, despite the best intentions of the person who refers you to an oncologist, you may find the choice does not sit well with you. The best course of action is to raise the matter early with the referring doctor or, of course, the oncologist herself. The daughter of a non-English-speaking patient found it unhelpful to see a different oncologist each time in the outpatient clinic of a public hospital. She felt that she spent most of her time bringing the new doctor up to date with her father's situation, which left little time to ask important questions. The process was necessarily slow due to the language barrier. After two such visits she brought it up with the oncologist who agreed to put a note in her file that he should be seen by the same doctor as much as possible. This arrangement worked for her father but two years later, when her mother developed cancer, the daughter took her to see a private oncologist who spoke her mother's language, thus removing the obstacles her father had faced.

A simple misunderstanding about why you are kept waiting or why your chemotherapy cannot always be delivered on the same day can be clarified, but when there are serious clashes of personality or a divergence of goals of care, it pays to consider other options. Keep in mind that no oncologist deliberately wants to create a disgruntled or unhappy patient. As a cancer patient, you have enough to worry about, and don't need the additional stress of skirmishes with the very person you have entrusted your health to. Some of my patients seek a second opinion when they are not sure about my advice. When patients are upfront about their need, I facilitate their request by supplying relevant documents and writing to the new doctor, who is then able to provide an informed opinion. Some patients feel reassured and return to my care but some also leave. Like most oncologists, I don't mind as long as the patient is well served. A dissatisfactory doctor–patient relationship is not in anyone's interest. In some public clinics patients can ask to see a particular oncologist they feel comfortable with. Sometimes they refuse to see anyone else even if this means the wait is twice as long. 'Doctor, I don't mind seeing you, but is it okay if I wait for my usual doctor?' a patient asks. Thus put, it is difficult to take offence; instead, it's good to see that there is someone the patient trusts and who knows the patient well. This is not unusual. As I have noted, patients look to an oncologist for emotional support as much as medical facts – it's natural that each patient will find a different fit with a doctor.

Sometimes it is not until further along the course of treatment that a patient realizes the need for a different oncologist. This may be because your initial goals were aligned, but they no longer are. A friend of mine found that once his mother's cancer progressed beyond treatment, her oncologist was unwilling to engage in a conversation about prognosis. Increasingly, this meant that she was enduring toxic treatment without adequate information on which to base her decision. He finally convinced her to see a second oncologist who spoke more openly about maximizing quality of life by avoiding futile chemotherapy. Her mother later said that this was the most informative and therapeutic conversation she had had in all her time as a cancer patient. Patients commonly believe that if one doctor possesses their medical history, it is difficult for this to be transferred. My friend's mother feared the same, but in fact the second oncologist did not need every minutiae of her treatment to understand the broad picture and provide a meaningful discussion about her future. The second oncologist corresponded with the first and this was all it took for the original oncologist to become involved with the patient again. My friend's mother ended up staying with the original oncologist because he was closer to home, but felt happier with their subsequent conversations.

Of course, not everyone can handle changing oncologists, and not everyone needs to; indeed, it may not be possible. But there are ways to get the most out of your consultation. It is okay to set out your expectations with your oncologist. These may include your wanting written information from time to time, asking permission to jot down important conversations you wish to think over at home, bringing a trusted relative to every consultation, or sometimes handing over a set of written questions to jog your memory. You may be somebody who likes to look at your medical scans or save copies of your results, or you may be happy to leave them to the oncologist. Like most people, oncologists respond well when they know what you expect of them, so don't be afraid to ask and negotiate.

It is also important to learn what your oncologist is like. By all means, ask questions firmly and politely about your treatment, without being unnecessarily confrontational. He may need prior warning through his secretary that you are coming in to discuss the cessation of treatment or that you need an urgent insurance claim filled out. Don't assume that your oncologist always has test results at hand – you may need to ask in advance about them. Accept the occasional wait with good humour, recognizing that the most likely reason for the delay is the unanticipated needs of someone before you, and that you may be that patient one day. Being sharply demanding may get you results the first time or two, but being good-natured and gracious tends to win in the end.

Your relationship with the oncologist is a partnership. Like all partnerships, it will take time, effort and understanding, and perhaps an element of luck. Don't expect it to be perfect but it should meet your most important needs. If not, trying someone else may be the answer. Mostly, you should feel like a genuine partner in your treatment, a participant not a passive observer.

Key Points

- An oncologist is a specialist physician who prescribes chemotherapy and monitors the course of your cancer and undergoes years of rigorous training and assessment.
- Your relationship with the oncologist is prolonged; so it pays to find someone you respect, trust and can talk to. It's okay to take some time to find the right oncologist.
- When choosing an oncologist be mindful of practical concerns around your decision, such as cost, logistics and support structures because they will become increasingly meaningful with time.
- Being a partner in your treatment means setting reasonable expectations of communication with your oncologist and ensuring that they are met.

5

What to Expect When Having Chemotherapy

I recently reviewed the treatment of an eighty-four-year-old man with advanced bowel cancer. When I first met him, he had been undergoing investigations for three months. Although inconvenient, this had not proven detrimental to his health. This fact, and the knowledge that his scans did not reveal incipient danger, reassured me that chemotherapy was not urgent. He suffered from heart disease but was otherwise a relatively fit man who still mowed his lawns and painted his fence. He was happily married to an equally fit and active wife and together they enjoyed the retirement they had long envisioned when they ran a busy convenience store.

In fact, the question I had in my mind during our initial meetings was whether he ought to have chemotherapy at all, because his disease was incurable but indolent and I wanted to spare him the expected toxicity of treatment. Given his age, I wondered whether the cancer would necessarily affect his lifespan before his heart or another organ caused trouble. But mindful of the propensity of doctors to undertreat many elderly people and the widespread perception that the very elderly population faces discrimination, I wanted to be careful not to dismiss chemotherapy altogether, especially if he wanted it. As it turned out, both the patient and his wife were extremely eager to have the cancer treated and became irritated at my perceived delay in organizing it. The patient was provided with written and oral instructions about the side effects to expect. He made a thinly veiled comment about the length of time it had taken doctors to get moving. Finally the day arrived when he started chemotherapy, the mildest effective version I could prescribe to test his tolerance before I escalated treatment. He did so well that I began to chastise myself for having doubted his robustness. Alas, the honeymoon did not last long and soon he was back in my office.

'You didn't tell it would be like this,' he started.

'Tell me how you are,' I replied, although his response was already painted on his face.

'The chemo itself is okay but I hate the travel, the waiting, the needles and the terrible fatigue that sets in afterwards.'

'We thought the chemo would be quick but it takes hours,' his wife added, clearly feeling the pressure too. 'The other day, he needed another blood test, which added three hours to our wait.'

As I listened to their complaints, I felt sympathetic and a little frustrated at the situation. Over two education sessions they had been advised, warned and prepared for the journey ahead. It was tempting to rebut all of their claims by saying, 'We told you so', but the fact is no one quite knows how the theoretical talk about chemotherapy applies to them until they have experienced it. However, it was also clear that they had been subject to so much information overload that they had tuned out. They had filed away the written information without reading it and couldn't recall anything from the education session. 'It was one big blur because, to be honest,' the man said, 'I just wanted to get on with the chemo.'

If you are about to undergo chemotherapy you are probably spending a lot of time wondering what to expect. Having accompanied numerous patients on their varied journeys through the treatments, I see that a significant part of how you experience chemotherapy depends on the expectations you carry into it. Certainly, there are unexpected events that can catch us all by surprise, but I want to spend some time discussing some standard expectations of chemotherapy.

Let us start on a positive note. People will be nice to you! Whether it is the passenger riding in the train with you, the stranger in a common waiting room, the frantic emergency department doctor or the harried pathology nurse, you will notice that your situation invokes kindness. You might be tempted to doubt that kindness at times. 'No one cared about me at work until I had cancer, and now it feels like the whole office is my best friend,' a young woman once reported, a little cynically.

When her law firm had been coping with a major financial setback, she was subjected to some harsh assessments and only just retained her job. Soon after, she was diagnosed with cancer. 'As the newest graduate, I was an easy target, but when I got cancer, everyone suddenly felt guilty and wanted to make it up to me.' She was probably accurate in that everyone did feel a bit guilty.

Nonetheless, others are simply touched by a patient's plight and want to do anything possible to help. Doctors, nurses and other professionals enter this field of medicine because they feel a special affinity towards cancer patients. My advice is to not second-guess people's motives too much and accept that their behaviour towards you may indeed be softened by your diagnosis. When someone we know has cancer we are sobered by the knowledge, because their diagnosis feels like a brush with our own mortality. It is okay, then, to accept kindness and compassion without feeling patronized. I know that I often go the extra length for my cancer patients because I feel their needs are more acute. I may sound more solicitous towards them, but this is not to diminish their autonomy. Rather it is because I care deeply about them. So if people are nice to you, accept it gladly.

But what to expect from the treatment itself? Cancer therapy includes chemotherapy, targeted therapy and hormonal therapy. None of these treatments is benign, but chemotherapy typically causes the most side effects; so I want to devote particular time to it here.

Although we would like to selectively destroy the cancer cells and leave normal cells untouched, chemotherapy inevitably affects normal cellular structures too; so it is usual for patients to experience a range of side effects. The commonest of these include nausea, vomiting, hair loss, infection risk and fatigue. You may experience very little of these effects or experience some of them intensely depending on the type of chemotherapy, your general health and your sensitivities. You will find that your doctor or nurse will routinely ask you about a handful of side effects and suggest appropriate management, which may include drugs as well as modification to your treatment. Chemotherapy can result in a broad range of problems that range from a mild annoyance to serious threats to life. The latter category, such as a dangerous fall in kidney function, a life-threatening infection or significant anaemia, tends to be identified and corrected quickly, but even the niggling problems can impair your quality of life. It helps to be aware of a plethora of side effects that are perhaps not as commonly discussed, which can result in a situation where the patient might simply keep quiet about them and miss out on their possible correction. At some point in your treatment, preferably early, I recommend reading through the side effects, which can be provided to you. This way, if you do experience something that was not mentioned in your consultations, you are aware that it can still be related to the therapy, and potentially counteracted.

Chemotherapy means travel. Whether you are receiving intravenous chemotherapy (the most common forms, involving a 'drip' inserted into a vein) or oral (increasingly in use, involving pills) you will have many appointments to keep. Most patients completely underestimate the amount of travelling they will need, and not just to chemotherapy appointments but also to visit their oncologist, their GP, the pathology and radiology suites, the pharmacy and so on. Of course these are just the essentials. You may also need to fit in periodic appointments to your surgeon, other specialists, the dentist, physiotherapist, dietician and welfare benefits offices, not forgetting that everyone wants to preserve a modicum of a personal and social life to feel normal. Travel is expensive and time-consuming. Much of it requires someone else to accompany you, with implications for their time management too. Even if prolonged travel does not bother you initially, it will catch up with you eventually, especially if you expect to become unwell with time and are likely to receive prolonged therapy. This is why it is very important to seek treatment close to where you live, unless there are special circumstances that entail you bypassing locally based care. I meet many patients who choose somewhere further away from home than necessary because they believe that a more prestigious cancer centre always means better care. As I have explained before, if you have an uncommon cancer or you are undergoing a special treatment not widely available such as through a clinical trial, you may need to find a specialized centre, but if you live in a metropolitan area, or a large regional town with a cancer centre, the chances are that you can receive good treatment and care right where you are, thus saving you and your carer a lot of travel. Even if you have begun receiving therapy further afield but now wish to move closer to home, don't let fears of the paperwork necessary stop you from arranging the move. Doctors and nurses are proficient at chasing up past details and will put your needs first.

Chemotherapy also involves long waits. This will happen in all the places that I have mentioned above. Everyone is sympathetic to cancer patients and you will receive priority assistance when possible, but the truth is that with the number of cancer patients on the rise you will almost certainly find that your needs are not always met as quickly and efficiently as you would like. You will find yourself enduring many periods of idleness. These may be in the waiting room to see your oncologist, in the chemotherapy chair waiting for your treatment to be hooked up, waiting to have a blood test or a scan, or waiting, often nervously, for results of various tests. It is unfortunately likely that at some point you will get sick of the sitting around and become irritable at your providers for keeping you waiting.

I recently called in on a patient at exactly 10 a.m., her scheduled appointment time. 'What?' she exclaimed, nearly spilling her drink. 'I just sat down with my first coffee and a book! I come prepared to wait the first half-hour, and then another half depending on who has gone in before me.' The wait matters to her because she still works and having her consultation later translates into a later treatment time, which results in her needing the day off for what is only a thirty-minute infusion. Although she was smiling pleasantly, she was expressing how she has resigned herself to waiting in clinic – a punctual appointment took her by surprise. She has often expressed puzzlement at why oncologists, or for that matter all doctors, run late. Like most, I am a punctual professional and see my first patient as scheduled, but it is sadly true that by the time the last patient of the day has been seen, appointment times often bear little resemblance to the schedule.

If you have ever wondered why this happens, let me provide an account of a typical morning that might lead to such delays.

I see the first patient and our consultation takes the scheduled fifteen minutes. In the midst of our discussion, I receive a phone call from a lawyer who has filed a claim for asbestos-inflicted disease for my mesothelioma patient and wants to obtain an urgent statement of his prognosis. I promise to send him a report by the end of the week, before bringing in my next patient. This patient reports complicated pain that takes a long time to address. Multiple prescriptions and their regulatory approval take time. The patient's wife is also concerned about his diet and it seems rude to cut her off in the hope of finding time to discuss it another day. This consultation extends to thirty minutes. The next patient is wheelchair- bound and it takes her extra time to simply make her way into my room and settle herself in a comfortable spot. Having suffered a stroke, she is slow to move, speak and understand. But she is reasonably well from her cancer and our consultation keeps to time. The patient after her is an African refugee, frightened, vulnerable and very unwell. By the time I find an interpreter, decipher her symptoms and formulate a plan of care, I have gone past the appointments of two other patients. I think you get the idea. Cancer is an illness that comes with multiple complications, and sometimes unpredictable ones that are only unearthed at the time of the appointment. Pre-allocating a long slot to every patient would simply slow down the whole process. So by necessity, appointment windows tend to be kept short. We anticipate some patients will require less time and others will need more than their allotment.

If you experience a delay in the delivery of your chemotherapy it may be because many of the agents in the treatments themselves are prepared on the day, after your oncologist gives the go-ahead. Pre-packed chemotherapy can still be delayed if the oncologist alters the orders after reviewing your symptoms. Of course, you want to have the treatment tailored to your current situation, but unfortunately this might take some time. A doctor or nurse may flag your blood test as urgent but in a large hospital there are many competing problems of this magnitude. So although it may seem strange that an urgent result takes two hours, that may be considered a fast turnaround in a bustling service.

I hope these explanations might help you appreciate that despite the best intent, your wait can be caused by circumstances beyond the control of your medical carers. And remember, of course, that you might require an extra-long consultation yourself one day, when you present yourself sicker and more vulnerable than you ever thought you could be. So be prepared to wait, as much as possible with good grace. Bring a good book, a good friend, a snack, pain relief or whatever it is that you find helps you pass time. Indeed, if you have friends who have asked how they can help, suggesting that they accompany you to chemotherapy could be a good idea. It makes them feel useful and provides a way for you to be distracted throughout any delays.

If your wait is consistently uncomfortable, inconvenient or unacceptable for another reason, do bring it up with the staff. A recent patient had to battle heavy Monday morning traffic to reach the clinic for a scheduled appointment that was rarely on time. Unbeknown to us, she had moved to a rural town to live with her son, which made the journey even more arduous. Upon discovering her problem, we shifted her appointment to a more convenient time when traffic had settled. Another patient could not sit for long in a hard chair because of back pain. We started giving him the first appointment of the day. If you don't bring up the delay with your doctor or nurse you won't know if there is a way to fix the problem. Here, nurses, in particular, can be a great ally.

The process of receiving chemotherapy is uncomfortable for many and painful for some. Many people experience what we call anticipatory anxiety in the days or hours leading up to chemotherapy (others may experience a more pervasive form of anxiety or depression, which I'll discuss in a later chapter). One of the uncomfortable factors is the insertion of an intravenous line. Some people can find it a traumatic experience. One patient recently said, 'I don't mind it once the chemo starts but it's the lead up to it that I hate. I used to have good veins, but with time they have been used up and it's always an anxious time to see how many attempts it will take for someone to find a vein.' Many patients describe becoming resigned to being routinely stuck by sharp needles. Some people opt for a more permanent line, which can be accessed by a nurse to give chemotherapy or take blood. This is placed under local or general anaesthetic, but these are not without complications either. If you have one of these more permanent intravenous access sites, usually located in your elbow (a PICC, which stands for a peripherally inserted central catheter) or your upper chest (a port, also known as a port-a-cath), infection and clotting can be an issue. Regular care in the form of flushing or dressing change is required to avoid complications, and that usually means more travel.

A chemotherapy unit, in a private or public hospital, is typically filled with activity. While it is not an outright boisterous place, and there is a genuine attempt to protect your need for quiet space and rest, you should not expect it to be an oasis of calm. There is a lot of traffic as patients are treated and discharged to make way for newcomers. Occasionally, there are also confronting sights of patients looking upset, unwell or undergoing a reaction to chemotherapy. You may overhear conversations. The staff will always try to shield you from other people's unpleasant experiences but in a confined space it is inevitable that you will notice things you don't like. On the other hand, you may also make friends while having chemotherapy, especially if you meet the same few patients on fixed days. Some patients are wary of others, or feel awkward speaking to strangers about such a personal subject as cancer treatment – it is okay if you are one of them and prefer to read, listen to music or just talk to your friend. But others will share a word with their neighbour and carers may befriend each other. There is enormous support to be found for some people in these interactions, which normalize their own experience. Some time ago I wrote about two patients, of differing ages, religion and life experience, who sat in adjoining chemotherapy chairs. They became friends and helped each other through some difficult times. When one died, the other felt very sad but was also heartened to hear how much he had helped his new-found friend in coping with illness. My advice to you is that there is no protocol for how you must spend your time in the chemotherapy chair – do what feels right to you each time.

While having chemotherapy, you will typically not need an involved consultation with your oncologist on every occasion, but you will always be supervised by a nurse who has access to one. If a nurse needs assistance with something straightforward, such as writing a prescription, or reviewing a sore throat or a painful leg, a junior doctor may be called upon. Junior doctors know to escalate their concerns to a senior colleague if needed. Every chemotherapy unit has a protocol of contacting the oncologist over serious matters. For example, a nurse may consider it unsafe to administer chemotherapy if she suspects you are critically unwell. Or the nurse may uncover that you are struggling with the side effects of chemotherapy without anyone having fully appreciated the extent of your trouble. You may occasionally find that a junior doctor and a nurse have differing views on how to treat you and your oncologist is asked to clarify things. Sometimes this will result in a change of plan, which could be as substantial as you not receiving chemotherapy as planned. Don't be put off by these events – they are happening with your best interest in mind, and are the result of several professional people working out how best to care for you. Remember to speak up and ask to be reviewed by a doctor if you are feeling unsure about something.

Most patients feel okay in the immediate aftermath of chemotherapy because of the potent drugs given at the time to prevent acute nausea, vomiting and so on. One patient put it this way: 'After dreading the whole thing, I was thrilled when nothing bad happened for the first three days. But later that week, I felt very ordinary and tired, although thankfully, nothing terrible happened.' Another patient did not experience any of the mentioned side effects of chemotherapy but two weeks after taking an oral chemotherapy pill experienced serious mood swings resulting in road rage. He did not deem himself safe to drive and ended up switching treatments with good effect.

You might find that your oncologist advises you not to pronounce on your experience of chemotherapy too early, especially if the early side effects are being ironed out with better supportive management such as stronger anti-nausea pills, injections to boost your white cell count and the like. While your patience may be required as the team works towards optimizing your care, do speak up about alarming or unacceptable side effects that will only cause harm if not addressed immediately.

Generally, you will begin to recognize a pattern in how your body handles chemotherapy. Some people feel okay in the first few days after chemotherapy before some of the short-term drugs wear off and side effects settle in. Other people feel particularly unwell in the initial days and then get progressively better. I find that a person's experience of the first few cycles provides a fair indication of what to expect in the short term. But chemotherapy also has many cumulative toxicities, falling blood counts and fatigue being two common ones which become apparent after several cycles.

Other things to expect during chemotherapy include information overload. Keep a notepad at hand and don't ever hesitate to ask for a repeat explanation. Expect that you will not understand the precise importance of everything to do with your cancer, but with patience, assistance and being gentle with yourself, you will get there.

Finally, be prepared for a change of plans. Cancer is an extraordinarily wily disease that defies expectations, and you may find your oncologist wanting to change course midway through planned therapy. This may be guided by new knowledge, better drugs or a better understanding of your situation. Don't take this as a reflection of anything other than your doctor's interest in your welfare. Try to be open to changes in the plan. Just in the past few weeks I have witnessed some striking unexpected occurrences. A ninety-year-old patient of mine who came to the hospital with severe anaemia and renal failure, after sustaining a fall at home, miraculously survived our grim predictions and is now home again. He is walking, reading the newspaper and entertaining his family. His prostate cancer is the least of his problems. But a young woman with advanced breast cancer became unwell in the week prior to starting chemotherapy and her condition deteriorated very quickly, leading to a hasty change of plans. One man's liver disease disappeared with treatment, eliminating the need for an operation, while his cousin took to a wheelchair from an unprecedented severe reaction to what is usually considered a safe drug. What these cases illustrate is that despite our diligence, oncologists are simply not able to predict everything you can expect from chemotherapy. Coping with uncertainty is an integral part of having cancer, and bolstering your resilience is very helpful. I hope that the upcoming chapters of this book will help you better understand many aspects of cancer, because a good understanding goes hand in hand with the ability to cope.

Key Points

- Chemotherapy refers to cancer treatment that is delivered in a number of ways although most commonly via an intravenous drip.
- Chemotherapy is a complex treatment that has many side effects. Short-term effects are different from longer-term ones. Although you may not understand all the moving pieces, aim to understand some of the most important toxicities and what to do about them for treatment to proceed smoothly.
- There is always a degree of uncertainty involved in cancer management, but asking the right questions can help reduce it.
- Eventually, many confusing things will become routine, you will settle into a pattern and know what to expect.

6

Deciding Whether to Have Treatment and Understanding Side Effects

In the throes of your anxiety about the future or your enthusiasm to just get started with treatment so that you can beat the disease, you might regard this chapter curiously. After all, what's there to decide about having treatment for a condition as serious as cancer? As more than one patient has scoffed, 'I will die without treatment, so what's the decision here?' I hate to imagine that my patients think I am frittering away their time with indulgent questions that they can ill afford to ask. But this is an emerging question in many areas of medicine, not all cancer-related: What is the net benefit of a treatment that is usually accompanied by side effects? For some the benefit is clear. They are being treated with the intention of cure, which means that the inconvenience of temporary side effects may be worth the long-term chance of being free of disease. But for many people, especially those with advanced or metastatic (and hence typically incurable) forms of illness, or conversely, very early cancer, if we agree that one of our goals is to maximize the quality of life by avoiding significant toxicity, this is an important question to ponder. Like many patients, you might be feeling too frightened or overwhelmed to give this matter much thought, but I think it is worth your time.

I want to start by telling you about a memorable patient, Peter. Everyone wants to own him as a patient – the surgeon, the radiation doctor and the oncologist. But in a polite way, Peter dislikes medical professionals, and given half a chance, is quick to espouse the view that the secret of his well-being is his successful avoidance of doctors.

At eighty-two years of age, Peter was diagnosed with early prostate cancer via a blood test that his doctor obtained as part of his annual check-up. Scans and a biopsy followed and a multidisciplinary team concluded that with his type of early prostate cancer, there was no so-called 'best' treatment. Rather, there were options, and it would come down to an informed decision taken by the patient. Armed with the phrase he had heard most often in the past few weeks – 'patient preference' – he did the round of doctors to see if they could help him decide.

The urologist kept Peter waiting for two hours as he was caught up in theatre. Finally, the surgeon arrived and ushered (or as Peter described it, *herded*) him in. He was a man in his forties who worked at a flying pace. Everything from the surgeon's illegible writing to his advice was rushed and he made no attempt to curb it. The prostate cancer was early and hence operable; Peter could have the operation next week. The procedure was reasonably straightforward, he performed a few every day, and the outcome was usually good. 'But there is a risk that you could end up with impotence or incontinence and ...' At that point, Peter lost interest. When his wife, Elizabeth, asked him later what the surgeon said, all he could reply was, 'I don't think the operation is necessary, love.' In his mind he thought that even if it was, that surgeon wasn't the right man for him. He wanted someone with more time.

Peter's doctor arranged for a second opinion from an older surgeon. He didn't think that surgery was essential but spoke about suppressing the male hormone testosterone that encouraged prostate cancer growth. But along with the names of drugs, he rattled off another list of side effects that seemed no less daunting than the surgery's. Peter heard 'impotence, hot flushes, heart and bone disease' and thought that if it were up to him, he would just collect his spade and shears and get right back to gardening. But Elizabeth would worry, so he felt he had to try harder.

Next on the list was the radiotherapy doctor. She was a pleasant Irish lady and they spent a bit of time talking about his youth in Ireland. She told him she could offer radiotherapy but it too had a variety of side effects, some long-lived. Peter's thoughts went immediately to his friend Barney, who suffered persistent diarrhoea and the urge to urinate following radiotherapy for prostate cancer. What could be worse than running to the toilet every hour while he was tending his garden? He heard that the radiotherapy would happen every day for a few weeks. Who would run his business if he was constantly in and out of hospital? Elizabeth could manage for a few hours or days but not weeks. She couldn't keep track of where the various plants were, and hated doing large orders. It didn't take long for Peter to cross out radiotherapy as an option, but he couldn't bring himself to tell the doctor just yet. So he asked for some time to think it over. In actual fact, he was going to use that time to plant a long-promised rose garden for an old friend.

As he enjoyed getting his hands dirty in the soil, he noted to himself that the two surgeons and the radiation doctor were equally confident about their recommendations. Could it be possible that both treatments were similarly effective? And if so, why didn't anyone say so clearly? Why did one expert pit his opinion against another? The final doctor on his list was the oncologist, which was me. With delays and cancellations, it had taken him two months since diagnosis to get through his list of doctors. I could tell that he was impatient to cover the last base. 'I know that surgery is not for me, neither is radiotherapy. I have talked to my GP, Dr Joe, about hormones to block testosterone and I can't say they sound too good either. Hot flushes, impotence, heart problems are just the ones I remember.' He fixed with me an earnest gaze. 'Tell me doc, is it really necessary to have any treatment?' I looked at him curiously. Usually the question from patients is about how much treatment, not whether to have any.

'I have some graphs and figures I can show you that help predict the risk of the cancer spreading – would it help if you saw them?' I offered.

He simply answered, 'No, I want to trust someone to be straight with me.'

All doctors make decisions about their patients – whether to try one drug or another, whether to recommend surgery or not, whether to even bring up the possibility of certain therapies that may disappoint or are unaffordable. But somehow, the recommendation whether to have or forgo cancer treatment seems particularly weighty and in a different class altogether. I think it's because the subject of mortality never strays too far from the mind when one mentions cancer. Starting or stopping someone's aspirin or blood pressure tablet may well have serious long-term consequences, but if you get cancer therapy wrong, the results can be acutely distressing and potentially fatal. So it is always with a heightened sense of respect and responsibility that I take on a patient's request for me to judge what is best for them.

As I listened to Peter however, I was consoled that he had long made his decision – he was just looking for an oncologist to back him up. It was clear that Peter's life revolved around his ability to be in his nursery and garden. He was indefatigable in the garden and was very clear that he wanted to be in a healthy state for as long as possible.

'Peter', I advised, 'if you were much younger, there could be an argument to act now, because of the potentially longer lifetime over which the cancer could grow and spread. But at eighty-two with early prostate cancer, you can afford to wait and watch.'

'When I first found out, of course I wanted something done about it,' he said. 'But the more people I talked to, the more I realized that nobody was offering me a free cure. There are serious problems associated with whatever you do – I'm damned if I do and damned if I don't. I'm a simple man, doctor. I just don't think the risk is worth taking, not at my age.'

'What does Elizabeth say?'

'She says to get back to the job and stop wasting everyone's time if I've made up my mind!'

'Peter, let me ask you something. Does uncertainty bother you? I mean the uncertainty of relying on your instincts, when experts around you are recommending their treatment.'

'No. All my life I have trusted my gut feeling.'

'I wish more people could put as much trust into their instinct as you do.'

'I've listened carefully to all the doctors. Now, no one is saying I *must* have treatment. What they are saying is that treatment is available. I reckon they're two different things.'

I was struck by the astuteness of a man who would rush to describe himself as simple and unsophisticated. Thanks to decades of painstaking work, there is plenty of good evidence in oncology about things that work and don't work. But scientific data is nuanced and should be interpreted as liberally or conservatively as you like. Should an operation be done simply because it is technically feasible? Is a six-week increase in survival due to chemotherapy significant? It depends. To a thirty-year-old mother of three, every day counts. To the octogenarian ailing widow, perhaps not. Would you be willing to exchange greater toxicity, including, say, vomiting, fatigue or infection risk, for a potential gain in life? Again, it depends on the value you place on quality versus quantity. If you are twenty-four years old, that gain could mean a lot. If you are sixty-four, you may just think about it a little more. But at ninety-four you might dismiss the proposal completely. So decisions about chemotherapy are not always about right or wrong, black or white, as much as living by a personal philosophy, elements of which change with age.

The next week I sat down with Peter and his wife to reassure her that he had not made a rash decision but an informed choice. I made arrangements to see Peter in a few months' time. I told him that if he wanted, I could do an occasional PSA test (PSA stands for Prostate Specific Antigen, a blood test used to monitor prostate cancer)and we could always revisit his decision. He seemed happy with this degree of control and on his way out told the secretary that he was delighted at the reprieve. He had not slept the previous night thinking that I would change my mind.

That was six years ago. Peter is now eighty-eight, completely well, and still working hard in his nursery. He has had to hire an extra hand – his eldest grandson, who takes after his grandfather. Two years after his initial diagnosis, Peter decided that he didn't want to have his PSA checked at all. 'I feel fine and I'm not interested in knowing what a number is doing,' he declared. It was hard to argue with his logic.

It seems that like many older men, Peter will die *with* and not *of* prostate cancer. He still comes to see me, joking that he does so as a public service reminder that all cancers do not equate to doom. When I see him I can't help thinking that his life could have been significantly adversely affected by the proposed treatment. Peter is a good example of taking ownership of one's health decisions. No one could have predicted the precise effect of therapy on Peter, but he himself was always sure about one thing – he wanted to be the chief decision maker. This is not an easy role to assume, but for those who do it successfully, it can be a rewarding one.

Patients like Peter who are diagnosed early with the disease are lucky to avoid toxic treatment, but there are many others who are found to have metastatic disease, that is, cancer that has spread beyond the initial site, and for whom chemotherapy would be a usual recommendation. Perhaps you are in this situation, where you are expecting to have chemotherapy. But you may be wondering whether it is right for you. How do you know that you will tolerate it well, and moreover, derive benefit? And what will the benefit look like? Perhaps you wonder whether you will eventually be healthier and live longer.

The diagnosis and staging of cancer are relatively straightforward compared to the decision about treatment options. Thirty or forty years ago, treatment options were as woefully limited as our knowledge of how cancer behaves. Chemotherapy was available for only for a few diseases, and it was ruthlessly toxic. One of my retired bosses recalled sedating patients to enable them to tolerate treatment. If initial chemotherapy failed and the patient survived, there was the occasional option of a second-line drug, but it wouldn't be uncommon to accept that there was nothing else. Incidentally, palliative care as we know it today was yet to take shape; so even the comfort care was basic, relying on sympathetic words and gestures more than carefully studied therapies to alleviate suffering.

But in the last decade or so, medical knowledge has exploded, leading to ongoing advances in the design of new therapies. As a result, there is a profusion of treatments, and if you take into account various clinical trials being conducted around the world, and the ubiquity of Internet-based information for the patient and the oncologist, the most common cancers have more treatment options than the average oncologist can utilize. If the only question asked is, 'Is there *any* chance that this treatment will help?' you will find the answer likely to be yes. Unfortunately, this answer is not really helpful.

Before we discuss whether any particular treatment is right for you, let's go over some of the common terminology. Standard or first-line therapy (whether involving chemotherapy, radiotherapy, hormonal therapy, targeted therapy or a combination of these) is one that has usually been rigorously tested on large numbers of patients and has been shown to make a significant difference in some specific parameters, such as the time to cancer recurrence, prolongation of life or a reduction in troublesome symptoms. In other words, there is evidence that it helps patients and it can be useful to know roughly how it will help you.

Second-line, third-line, fourth-line therapy and so on refer to a change in chemotherapy treatment after standard therapy is deemed to have failed. The failure may be due to progression of the cancer or intolerable side effects, or a combination of causes. (Experimental therapies are those being studied on current cancer patients. These therapies are usually offered via a clinical trial or specialized access schemes run by drug companies. I will discuss them later in a separate chapter.)

Generally speaking, every time disease resists one line of treatment, the chances of responding to the next line are smaller because cancer cells are very good at developing new ways of resistance to drugs.

A medical oncologist's armoury contains three main weapons against cancer: chemotherapy, targeted therapy and hormonal therapy. Chemotherapy is the traditional form of treatment. The number of chemotherapy drugs currently outweighs targeted and hormonal therapies. It is also true that the vast majority of current cancer treatments utilize chemotherapy as the main treatment to which non-chemotherapy drugs can be added, although this might change in the future as more targeted therapies emerge.

Targeted therapies, virtually unheard of in clinical practice a few years ago, are becoming increasingly prominent. They are different from chemotherapy in important ways. Rather than the more blunt approach of chemotherapy, which broadly attacks cancerous cells, these therapies target specific internal pathways in dividing cancer cells. Traditional chemotherapy does more collateral damage to normal cells, which is why one experiences nausea, vomiting, hair loss and infections from it. Targeted therapies don't have the same severe side effects as chemotherapy, and are usually better tolerated. This doesn't mean that they are entirely without side effects. Many patients complain of a rash, nausea, diarrhoea or lack of appetite, and indeed, some targeted therapies can lead to life-threatening problems. Many targeted therapies are given in combination with chemotherapy, which exaggerates side effects.

Hormonal treatment is used for cancers that grow under the influence of hormones, such as breast and prostate cancer. Less frequently, they may also be used in other conditions. Contrary to popular belief, they too have side effects, but these are rarely life-threatening and patients are able to fashion a lifestyle to accommodate these effects.

Since chemotherapy is the backbone of most modern cancer treatments and its toxicities are the most dreaded, I want to use the next section to deal with decision making about whether or not to have chemotherapy.

There is a common saying that applies as much to medicine as it does to other aspects of life. If you go to a baker you will get bread and if you go to a butcher you will get meat. If you go to a complementary medical practitioner you will get vitamins and if you go to a chiropractor you will get manipulation treatment. Loosely speaking, in cancer treatment (oncology), a surgeon may recommend an operation, a radiation oncologist may recommend radiotherapy, and a medical oncologist chemotherapy. Competing recommendations usually occur where there is no straightforward solution. This is what happened recently when a patient of mine developed a recurrence of her cancer. The surgeon felt that the lump was small enough to remove. But the radiation doctor recommended first shrinking the tumour with a few weeks of radiation. Then someone suggested she should have chemotherapy too and sent her to me. The young woman had been through a very difficult time during her initial diagnosis and was adamant that she would not have more chemotherapy or another operation. When she told me frankly that the thought of further chemotherapy or surgery would plunge her into depression, as she'd experienced the first time, I knew that we had to avoid these two options. In the end, she received only radiotherapy, which worked well and provided a durable response, avoiding the need for an operation.

You may wonder how one diagnosis can attract such a variety of treatments. Surely one is superior to another and doctors should be able to decide which is best in a situation. But this is not necessarily true. Furthermore, every professional knows their area best and feels most confident recommending their form of treatment. The emergence of multidisciplinary teams in hospitals means that many experts weigh in on treatment to ensure that the patient receives optimal care. But it's well known that the availability of more options increases the risk of over-treatment.

If you are sent to a medical oncologist, your referring doctor thinks that you either require chemotherapy or should at least have a discussion about it. Oncologists, such as myself, don't necessarily intend to talk you into having treatment but prescribing chemotherapy is routine for them. The average oncologist sees hundreds of patients a year and a condition that seems unique to you is commonplace to them. This means that sometimes oncologists can unintentionally sidestep crucial information that you might expect us to broach. Minimizing harm is a good example – it has different meanings for doctor and patient. When discussing the side effects of chemotherapy, a busy doctor might tend to prioritize them into a hierarchy of what a patient most needs to know, which means perhaps emphasizing some side effects and skimming over others considered less important.

'You told me about infections and hair loss, but you never said the nausea would be so bad that I couldn't get out of bed,' a patient once reported tearfully. 'I have not been able to lift my head for the whole week. It's ten times worse than being pregnant.' I felt regretful that I had only mentioned nausea in passing while spending plenty of time on the remote risk of heart failure.

'The ringing in my ears is driving me insane,' said another. 'I can tolerate everything else but the ringing is like a shadow, following me day and night. I wish someone had told me it could be this bad because I would never have had chemotherapy.' This seventy-year-old patient unfortunately went deaf soon after abandoning his chemotherapy. His enjoyment of music disappeared and he became depressed. It's hard to know whether he would have had chemotherapy treatment if someone had emphasized the small but real chance of deafness, but the problem had a terrible impact on his life.

With the genuine improvement in cancer cure rates, many patients will be left to grapple with the sequelae of chemotherapy. It is very important, then, that any discussion of chemotherapy entails a detailed mention of side effects and the degree to which you should expect them. Although it is impossible to predict exactly how chemotherapy will affect you, an oncologist can make educated decisions based on your age, general health, stated preferences of what effects would concern you most and the proposed treatment itself. This is the only way in which you can decide which side effects are worth putting up with. For a diabetic on the verge of dialysis, any prospect of worsening kidney failure may be unacceptable, while for an actress hair loss may be the deal breaker. If you spend most of your time reading documents, diminished sensation in your fingertips may not be as objectionable as it would be to a concert pianist whose livelihood would be ruined if her fingers did not register the finest of touches. A woman with terrible memories of vomiting from her last chemotherapy twenty years ago could not bring herself to have any treatment that might lead to nausea, while an elderly man refused to have chemotherapy that might bring on diarrhoea and compound his existing problems with a colostomy bag.

This is a good place to mention that you should always try to take somebody with you to an appointment, especially those where key decisions are made. No matter how well and capable you feel, it is quite likely that a trusted escort will provide you support and add value to your recollection of the medical conversations you have.

Although the list of side effects from chemotherapy is daunting, modern medicine has made tremendous gains in handling many of them. Older oncologists speak of a time when they felt helpless about the severe nausea and vomiting that patients experienced, and their only recourse was to sedate patients. Now,with the advent of powerful anti-nausea drugs, those days are fortunately over. Over the years we have also learned how to better use antibiotics, painkillers, blood growth factors, transfusions and other measures to support patients through chemotherapy. When I mentioned this to a twenty-five-year-old nurse receiving chemotherapy for breast cancer, she looked at me in disbelief. Not having been out of pyjamas for a week after her first cycle, she could scarcely imagine that her peers twenty years ago might have suffered worse. Her plight highlighted the fact that despite major advances, chemotherapy-related toxicity is a major drawback to cancer treatment and one that can have enduring physical and psychological effects. So it is vital to be informed about what you are signing up for.

Many patients, of course, are courageously willing to brave intense toxicities for the sake of getting better. They may be self-motivated or be encouraged to do so by others. But the key question is, when should you soldier through side effects and when should you say enough is enough? 'I'm willing to go through this whole damn process, tough as it is, if you can tell me there's light at the end of the tunnel,' James, an electrician with malignant mesothelioma, recently told me. Mrs Jones, a seventy-six-year-old widow put it like this: 'Having chemo means a year out of my grandchildren's life – if I know that I can make up for it in the next five or ten years, I will do it, but if the answer is no, I really need to think carefully about whether to put up with it all.'

James and Mrs Jones are not unique in expressing the concern that undergoing the rigours of chemotherapy must make life substantially better than the alternative of forgoing it. This is a common sentiment – spoken and unspoken – in every patient's mind: 'Is it worth it?' Most people will want to know whether chemotherapy will help them live longer. Answers to that question can be interpreted in different ways: 'There's a reasonably good chance', for example, leaves room for different levels of confidence. Evaluating the risks involved in chemotherapy and its potential benefits – the risk-benefit ratio – is helped by the available statistics. And while again, no two patients, or for that matter, no two oncologists will interpret the numbers in exactly the same way, it is important for a patient considering chemotherapy to try to get his/her head around them. Stay with me as I quickly explain the paramount concepts of *relative* and *absolute* risk reduction.

Few people – including among oncologists – enjoy talking through statistics, but allow me to illustrate their benefit with a very simple example. Take a group of 100 patients with the same type and stage of your cancer. Without chemotherapy, ninety-eight will live and two will die in the next five years. With chemotherapy, ninety-nine will live and one will die. The *relative risk reduction* is 50 per cent, since the number of people who have been helped by having chemotherapy is one out of two. But the *absolute risk reduction* is 1 per cent, since only one extra person survived as a result of chemotherapy and ninety-eight people were destined to survive anyway. So one person out of 100 was helped by chemotherapy, but all 100 were exposed to the harms, some of which were immediately visible, others not. It is possible that one or two people out of the cohort of 100 might suffer fatal toxicity.

Here is a second example. Of the 100 patients with another cancer, fifty will survive and fifty die within five years. With chemotherapy, seventy-five will survive and twenty-five will die. The *relative risk reduction* is again 50 per cent, the same as the previous example, because where fifty patients would have succumbed to cancer, with the chemotherapy only twenty-five will. The *absolute benefit* is 25 per cent. This means that out of every 100 people to have chemotherapy, twenty-five will benefit, a much better figure than one out of 100. However, here too, all 100 will be exposed to potential harm.

A conversation with the oncologist in both scenarios may unfold like this:

'Doctor, what are the chances of chemotherapy helping in my situation?'

'Pretty good, actually. By having chemotherapy, you halve your chances of dying from cancer.'

To most people, this would sound like an appealing, even highly optimistic prospect. Studies have shown that patients are willing to accept much, much smaller gains in survival than 50 per cent.

But if the first question was followed up with further queries, the answers may give pause for thought.

'What does that actually mean for my condition?'

In the first scenario I described above, the answer is: 'Well, the figures show that roughly one out of every 100 people like you will live longer due to chemotherapy.'

But the answer in the second scenario is different: 'Studies show that out of every 100 people like you, twenty-five will live longer due to chemotherapy.'

So, although both chemotherapy treatments in these scenarios claim to halve your chance of dying, the true or *absolute* benefit gained is significantly different. For some patients, a one in 100 chance of a benefit is unfavourable and they would turn down chemotherapy outright in favour of enjoying quality of life without the side effects of treatment, and take a chance on survival. Some may consider a twenty-five in 100 chance of benefit unacceptable too, but others would conclude that having chemotherapy would put the odds in their favour. The key is that patients were able to make an informed decision.

Another way of explaining benefit is known as the *number needed to treat*; that is, statistically, how many patients need to have this chemotherapy before one of them is likely to receive a benefit? If chemotherapy is beneficial, you want the *number needed to treat* to be small. If chemotherapy has limited potential to help, lots of people will need to be treated before one patient sees a benefit, so the number needed to treat is high.

In the first example, the number needed to treat is 100 – this means that 100 patients need to have chemotherapy for one person to benefit – and hence the gain from chemotherapy is small. In the second example, the number needed to treat is four – only four patients need to be treated for one to gain – and hence the benefit is much larger.

Advances in cancer medicine mean that there are several good decision aids available to the oncologist to explain difficult concepts in simple terms with the help of words, numbers and graphs to suit different levels of comprehension. Part of understanding the numbers is appreciating when chemotherapy doesn't necessarily prolong life but is used to reduce the burden of cancer symptoms. It is true of many metastatic cancers that even the most aggressive chemotherapy does not buy any meaningful time; however, it may improve quality of life by alleviating symptoms, including pain, shortness of breath, coughing, headaches, weight loss and tiredness. This alone may make chemotherapy a worthy endeavour, provided the patient understands the difference between prolonging life and controlling symptoms. Thinking about these things may also help you choose between different types of chemotherapy, which might offer different absolute benefit along with their varied levels of toxicity.

Lara was a forty-nine-year-old patient of mine with metastatic cancer of the pancreas. When I met her I couldn't help noticing that she was spending a week of every month in hospital due to chemotherapy-related toxicity. Sometimes it was for a blood transfusion, other times for hydration. Some weeks her pain was awful, other weeks her bowels didn't work. I asked her why she was continuing to have chemotherapy and she snapped at me, 'For the same reason as everyone else – I want to live longer.' She was devastated to eventually realize that far from adding time to her life, chemotherapy might actually end it prematurely. At first she denied ever having been told this, but on closer reflection she said, 'I've been avoiding asking these tough questions, hoping the oncologist would find a way of letting me know if it was really bad.' When I advised that she should stop chemotherapy altogether, she was relieved that someone had made the decision for her. Far too many patients brave chemotherapy due to misconceived notions. They assume it will prolong their life or, even in the face of mounting evidence to the contrary, believe that they will eventually feel better. In some cases, it is indeed true that if you can withstand the rigours of chemotherapy you will stand to benefit, but often, this is not the case. Patients then believe that if things aren't looking up, their oncologist will surely let them know. But from an oncologist's viewpoint, a patient like Lara who looks comfortable with her own decisions, it's the right thing to keep giving chemotherapy until the patient says no more. After all, no one wants to paint a picture of doom and gloom if it isn't absolutely necessary. Despite good intentions, conversations about goals of care are unfortunately uncommon.

For some patients *any* plausible chance of benefit is worth the risk. Others value quality of life over everything else; still others want to know that they have done everything humanly possible to defeat the cancer. The frustrating thing for both patients and oncologists is that there really is no right or wrong answer. So when a patient asks me what I would do, I can't help feeling like a surly teenager when I answer, 'It depends.' To which they sometimes respond impatiently, 'Depends on what?'

To me, it depends on what you value. You might value the spirit and courage that have helped you in the past. You might have a gut instinct that you will beat the disease. You might value knowing within yourself that you fought a good fight. Or you might value an untainted quality of life for as long as possible, and the freedom from recurrent hospitalization, travel to the chemotherapy unit and blood tests. You might value taking the holiday of a lifetime or spending time with your children or grandchildren. You might not see the value in living longer if that life comes with complications, or you may feel that you have led a full life and don't fear death. Naturally, life is rarely simple, rarely an either-or situation. I believe facing decisions about cancer treatment is a time to act according to one's fundamental values.

Navigating one's values becomes easier when the medical information is complete. Research shows that patients presented with only *relative risk reduction* information are more likely to endorse chemotherapy – it sounds very promising expressed in this way – but they're also more likely to be dissatisfied with their decision, because they're left uncertain about what it means. When presented with further information, such as *absolute benefit* or *number needed to treat*, such patients are more likely to change their decision. If people clearly understand that chemotherapy will not prolong their life, they make different decisions to those who mistakenly believe it will. Of course it is equally important to understand if chemotherapy will prolong life because the information might buoy you in difficult times.

'I don't understand why you guys don't give that information in the first place', a sixty-two-year-old woman once grumbled, after having the risk and benefit evidence explained to her. She made a good point. Different oncologists explain what they are offering in different ways. Medical professionals don't intentionally withhold information, but far too many patients complain that they don't receive anywhere near as much information as they would like. I know that sometimes I'm not sure about the answers, and other times, despite the best of my efforts, a patient is not interested in having a conversation about numbers and statistics. Sometimes a patient prefers to trust me to do the right thing, and other times she has made up her mind well before she comes in to see me because there is no lack of advice, information and misinformation about cancer.

You may be at a point where you are really not sure about what to do. It's common to feel lost, but willing yourself to think through some options with a cool mind might save you future worry. Take some time to think of the things that matter most to you. Share these with your oncologist when deciding on treatment. Don't assume that they are personal things in your life that your doctor won't be interested in hearing – a good oncologist will be glad you are sharing your thinking with them, and will find it helpful in guiding you to the best treatment option. Perhaps together you can write out a list of things chemotherapy will and won't achieve. This is why it is so important to find an oncologist who you feel you can talk to. When you make a decision, you should feel it is an informed one.

Key Points

- Not every cancer requires immediate treatment and some cancers may never require toxic treatment. Doing nothing is a reasonable option sometimes.
- You cannot make a decision about the value of chemotherapy without having a frank and honest discussion about your priorities. This is especially relevant when your cancer is incurable.
- Central to your cancer management is understanding absolute and relative risk. Ask your oncologist to explain these to you in plain language using decision aids so that you can make informed decisions about treatment at this crucial time.
- Take a trusted carer or friend to any appointments that discuss major decision points. You may not remember everything that is said. Write down important information, request plain language explanations, and don't feel rushed into making a decision.

7

How Do I Know if My Chemo Is Working?

How often do you find yourself thinking this question as you make the trip to your next chemotherapy? Having invested much thought and emotion into entering chemotherapy, every patient's greatest hope is that it is all worth it.

If you have taken time off work, postponed important family events or wound up a business you'll naturally wonder if it was the right thing to do. Since having chemotherapy almost always involves the time of significant others, you also want to ensure that their time attending to you is well spent. Many of my patients say that they will push through chemotherapy if I assure them it is working. The slightest positive remark from the oncologist can sustain flailing spirits; the smallest negative connotation can cause tiny doubts to expand in the mind. Getting through chemotherapy is a critical double act where oncologist and patient must be in tune for things to succeed.

Before asking if chemotherapy is working, it's important to understand why you are having it. 'To save my life' is an obvious answer, but not all chemotherapy is given with that exact intent. It is common for patients to assume that all chemotherapy is roughly the same, which leads to concern when you're not doing as well as another patient you know. 'My cousin needed chemotherapy and finished two months ago but I am still going,' a patient recently said. 'Shouldn't we be getting the same treatment?' As it turns out, the only similarity was that both men had cancer. But their cancers were in different organs and required different durations of treatment.

I want to spend some time on important differences between types of chemotherapy to help you understand your situation better and be able to gauge how well your treatment is going.

Adjuvant chemotherapy is the name given to treatment following recovery from surgery. It is usually provided on the premise that any visible cancer has been surgically removed but there are certain features to suggest a high risk of cancer relapse, which can be lowered by chemotherapy. The risk of cancer relapse is estimated by considering many things about your cancer, including the pathology specimen (the cancerous tumour that has been removed), blood tests that might indicate microscopic cancer cells remaining in the bloodstream, genetic markers, age, personal and family history amongst others. You may be receiving adjuvant chemotherapy for the treatment of breast, bowel, lung or gynaecological cancer and your oncologist might have described its role as one of 'mopping up' invisible cells that if left behind can eventually lead to relapse. I have heard colleagues explain adjuvant chemotherapy as spraying the soil after pulling out the weed. Other cancers, such as pancreas, lung and gastric, as well as rarer varieties, might also warrant adjuvant chemotherapy after consideration.

The key aspect of adjuvant chemotherapy is that there is a prescribed course and time for its delivery. Your oncologist will advise you of the type of drugs and number of cycles you need. (Many patients find the terminology of chemotherapy confusing. A treatment plan refers to the broad direction of your treatment. It might include chemotherapy, surgery and other interventions. When speaking of chemotherapy, oncologists tend to use cycles and patients often speak in terms of courses, days or number of times.) A cycle of chemotherapy is usually followed by a break. A cycle might be two weeks on, one week off; one week on, one week off; once a month and so on. The most practical thing for you is to jot down the dates of chemotherapy – a doctor can work out the rest.

By the way, just as it is always a good idea to know what regular prescription medications you take, you should keep track of the chemotherapy you have had. The details will be helpful if you end up in an unfamiliar emergency department in a hospital, or you're seeking a second opinion, moving cities or changing doctors. While medical records are usually obtainable, it can take a long time and you will make life easier for yourself by having important details at hand, especially if you have had cancer treatment previously. Knowing the amount of chemotherapy you have had and when it was given can be helpful in assessing toxicity. I advise patients to keep a pocket diary in which they record the dates and, preferably, the names of all their cancer therapy. If, like many patients, you have blood tests and X-rays in different places, jot down when and where you had them so that any doctor can trace them in an emergency. These tasks only take a few minutes at a time, but being organized can make a tremendous difference someday.

While adjuvant chemotherapy is given with an intention to cure – that is, to help prevent cancer recurrence and hopefully prolong survival – palliative chemotherapy is for cancer that is usually advanced and cannot be got rid of. Some patients with advanced cancer might still undergo surgery to remove a tumour that is causing or is expected to cause complications. For example, the surgeon might remove a large rectal cancer responsible for an imminent bowel obstruction, or fluid might be drained from your chest or abdominal cavity to relieve pressure. While such surgery helps avoid an acute problem,the entire disease can't be safely removed and palliative chemotherapy is required to tackle the problem.

Palliative chemotherapy can shrink disease to allow remission (when a cancer is visible but does not cause symptoms) and longer survival. Other times, it can improve symptoms such as pain, shortness of breath or a build-up of fluid, all resulting in a better quality of life but not necessarily a longer life. While palliative chemotherapy might not banish your cancer, there is a good chance of many therapies stabilizing disease for prolonged periods. This is one of the major accomplishments of modern therapies, which do not yet promise a cure but keep patients alive and well for a longer period of time. Oncologists and scientists hope to keep building on these stepwise improvements to better prognosis.

But keeping disease under check for long periods of time with the help of chemotherapy has potential down sides, not least that there might be no defined end to your treatment. As discussed earlier, the rationale for ongoing palliative chemotherapy should be a moving negotiation between you and your oncologist.

Aside from adjuvant and palliative chemotherapy, patients might also receive chemotherapy with or without radiation therapy, either in preparation for or following an operation. Treatment given before an operation is referred to as preoperative or neo-adjuvant therapy. Chemotherapy and radiation therapy offered as concurrent treatment (meaning at the same time) or sequential treatment (meaning one after the other) is usually given with the intent of reducing the size of a cancer to make it operable. However, an operation is not always possible or desirable and the recommendation may be to have the combined treatment without surgery. Neo-adjuvant therapies, including combined treatments (known as chemo-radiotherapy), have a defined course that your oncologist or radiation oncologist will describe.

If this is the first time you are hearing about the different possible roles of chemotherapy you can see why it is important that you understand the intention behind your treatment. This allows you to better understand how long you will need it, what the potential gains are and, most importantly, what detailed questions you might want to ask your oncologist.

I want to return now to the question of whether your chemotherapy is working, which is one of the most common questions I am asked. In the case of adjuvant therapy, where there is no visible disease but there are indications of a risk of relapse, the benefit of treatment cannot truly be quantified at the time. An obvious indicator of chemotherapy's effectiveness is whether it is reducing the size of a cancerous tumour. Obviously, then, after surgery has removed all visible signs of the tumour, successful post-operative treatment can't be measured in this way.

I sometimes explain adjuvant chemotherapy as taking out an insurance policy. You take it out to reduce or cover risk but it is not a complete guarantee against recurrence. If your cancer never comes back, it might well be due to the chemotherapy, but it's possible the cancer would not have recurred anyway. And the cancer may return despite having adjuvant chemotherapy, a possibility many patients don't appreciate. Since all chemotherapy is toxic, understanding the rationale behind adjuvant chemotherapy might make it easier to decide whether you want to tackle it and what to reasonably expect.

When patients ask whether adjuvant chemotherapy is worthwhile, what they are really asking is whether it will guard against recurrence. In other words, how much additional benefit does chemotherapy provide over not having any?

Take a simplified situation where a patient is deciding between treatment and no treatment. She is advised that six cycles of chemotherapy delivered over six months will reduce the risk of recurrence of a particular cancer by half. If she has an aggressive disease with a high risk of recurrence, say 50 per cent over the next five years, then reducing this risk to 25 per cent is significant. But if she has a good prognosis of cancer with just an estimated 2 per cent chance of recurrence, the same chemotherapy will only reduce her risk to 1 per cent. She might not consider it worth the ordeal.

Attempting to understand your individual risk of recurrence is critical to the decision about receiving chemotherapy. If you are in a poor-risk category, meaning that the chances of disease relapse are high without any chemotherapy, you might push on with treatment, but if you are in a good-risk category, where chemotherapy adds very little benefit to the overall situation, you might decide against having adjuvant chemotherapy. These days, there are increasingly sophisticated decision-making tools that help doctors determine the need for chemotherapy with more accuracy. These tools are not yet perfect but they will help you start a conversation with your oncologist about what's best for you. Don't hesitate to ask for a plain-language explanation of your chemotherapy and its benefits. The same kind of thinking applies to defined courses of preoperative chemotherapy. Since they are given with curative intent, their value can only be judged at a later time if the cancer does not come back. The decision to continue must be guided by how you feel and conversations with your doctor.

Palliative chemotherapy, received by a majority of cancer patients, is given for metastatic, that is, incurable disease. The aim is to preserve quality of life for as long as possible. Palliative chemotherapy doesn't have a fixed number of cycles, although oncologists will use their experience to set loose limits. For example, they might start with three cycles and see how you tolerate the treatment, whether the tumour responds, and how you feel about continuing. Then they might push on for another two or three cycles, till you get to another decision point, and so on. At least with visible disease and obvious symptoms it is easier to monitor whether chemotherapy is working or not, which is very important given that such chemotherapy can last from weeks to years. Certain patients, including those with breast, prostate, bowel and lung cancer can find their palliative chemotherapy extending for more than a year or two, with good results. This leads to an unforeseen problem. A patient asked me to fill out some welfare and insurance forms that required me to mention that her disease was terminal in order for funds to be released early. She came to see me in distress. 'Why didn't anyone tell me I was dying?' I was taken aback, and responded, 'We can't get rid of your cancer, but you are not dying. In fact, you're doing really well.' The patient was puzzled: 'Then why did my insurance form say that I'm terminally ill?'

Terminal illness is a term used to describe an illness that is not strictly curable. It does not mean that a patient is imminently dying; indeed, you may live well and long with a terminal illness. A few of my patients have been alive with spreading, low-volume cancer for close to ten years. Presumably the disease biology they are experiencing is less aggressive than usual, allowing them to lead a good quality of life despite having cancer. Indicating the presence of a terminal disease on official forms can mean that the patient's financial benefits are assessed or freed more quickly, which is one reason why your oncologist may recommend it.

Once, cancer was uniformly fatal. But thanks to modern therapies, some cancers are being converted from a fatal illness to a chronic disease that nevertheless requires lifelong treatment. Some of the drugs used are toxic while others do not interfere too much with quality of life. For example, patients with a blood disease called chronic lymphocytic leukaemia can remain well for many years on therapy. Many patients with metastatic breast and colon cancer are surviving beyond two years with modern therapies. My longest-surviving patient with metastatic lung cancer is alive five years after diagnosis, sadly a rare feat. A patient with pancreatic cancer, which is usually associated with a poor prognosis, has been well for two-and-a-half years.

If you're receiving palliative chemotherapy and wondering whether it is working, here are some things to consider. Do you feel better? What were the key symptoms that troubled you before starting chemotherapy? If you couldn't walk a block before getting breathless, can you walk longer now? If you were spending half your day in bed due to fatigue, has chemotherapy allowed you to be up and about more? Has your cough improved? Has your pain settled? These are some of the more obvious things that you as a patient can judge far more accurately than doctors. If you're *feeling* better on chemotherapy, it's probably doing you some good. But if you're spending several days at a time just recovering from palliative chemotherapy, or the symptoms you started with are worsening, your appetite and weight are falling, and you just can't see the benefit of chemotherapy, I am afraid that chances are you are right and that it isn't helping. On the other hand, adjuvant chemotherapy can also leave you feeling washed out, but if it is being given with the intent of improving survival or achieving a cure, your oncologist may encourage you to work around the side effects rather than stop treatment altogether.

While your subjective feeling on chemotherapy is vitally important, objective measures of the benefit of chemotherapy can be had from blood tests and scans. Your oncologist might follow what are called *tumour markers*, with rising or falling trends providing an indication of your treatment's progress. A variety of scans including ultrasound, CT and PET (position emission tomography) can also be used to measure response. It is ideal to have scans performed at one good centre where a radiologist can draw upon old scans for comparison. A report that says your tumour measures 5 centimetres is not as useful as one that also mentions it was 8 centimetres two months ago when you began chemotherapy. A report that mentions numerous cancer spots is not as useful as one that says there are many spots but the majority of them are very tiny and non-specific, and unlikely to be causing trouble. These details matter, so check with your oncologist regarding recommendations about where to have your scans done. Scans don't tend to change as quickly as results from blood tests, so they are usually done less often, typically at two to three months' intervals. Your oncologist might not change course based on the results of a single scan, but instead wait to observe the trend. For example, a scan might show slight progression of your cancer but you feel well and your blood tests are stable. In response, your oncologist might decide to hold tight for the time being. This is increasingly the case with some modern therapies, called targeted therapies, which are thought to apply the brakes on cancer. In that case, the X-ray appearance of your cancer may not look remarkably different, which is why your oncologist will rely on more than X-rays, such as your symptoms, to judge response.

Sometimes a scan's result sways the decision to stop chemotherapy. You may not have been feeling well for some weeks and are dreading the thought of further chemotherapy to compound your fatigue. A scan shows that in the past month the tumour has spread extensively. A discussion of the results may cement your decision to avoid more chemotherapy – as it is failing to stop the cancer – with a view to concentrating on preserving the quality of the remaining life. Most patients on chemotherapy have frequent blood tests to monitor anaemia, white cell count and other organ functions, which determine the chemotherapy dose. Again, a single abnormal test may not change management but the trend tells a story. If you need a blood transfusion every month, or your chemotherapy is frequently deferred due to fatigue, infection or other problems, it's time to review whether the ongoing chemotherapy is appropriate.

I hope you can now see why asking whether chemotherapy is working is dependent on your expectations and situation. In the case of adjuvant chemotherapy, understand that it is the extent of risk reduction in the long term that justifies the short-term toxicity. If your risk of relapse is very small, chemotherapy may have little to add; if you have high-risk features, it may be worth adhering to the programme, provided there are no unacceptable toxicities.

If you are receiving palliative chemotherapy, it is even more important to understand its intention. Contrary to popular belief, most of this kind of therapy is not given to prolong life but to improve symptoms. So if you're fortunate enough to experience minimal symptoms, or conversely, your symptoms are worsening from chemotherapy, talk to your oncologist about whether you should be having it. Many patients don't realize that there are perfectly good and far less toxic ways of managing their most troublesome symptoms. They feel trapped into having costly and harmful chemotherapy because they think it is the only way to stay well, but fortunately, with modern advances in symptom management and palliative care, it may be unnecessary.

With this understanding, and having put some thought into your own goals of care, make an appointment with your oncologist to specifically discuss this issue. Don't be afraid to ask direct questions, such as 'Will this chemo prolong my life?', 'What will happen if I stop chemotherapy or have a break?' and 'Is there something less toxic you can suggest?' Remember that these decisions are seldom all or nothing, and that the best outcome is one that is arrived at with negotiation and mutual understanding. Communication in this area is not as comprehensive as many patients might like, but asking direct questions of your oncologist is more likely to yield answers than expectant waiting. Clarifying misconceptions and learning more about the precise benefit of chemotherapy is an important aspect of putting yourself through treatment. The answer to 'Is my chemotherapy working?' lies in how you expect it to work and what it is supposed to achieve.

Key Points

- Understanding your individual risk of cancer recurrence is critical to your decision about having chemotherapy. Understand from the outset why you are receiving treatment. In incurable cancer, relief of symptoms is a worthy goal.
- Ask at the beginning how your response will be measured, for example, by symptoms, scans or blood tests. Usually, more than one of these is used. The question of whether chemotherapy is working for you relies on understanding your own expectations within the context of your illness.
- Periodically reviewing your goals of chemotherapy helps cast a light on whether the toxicities of treatment are still worthwhile enduring and,if so, how you might manage them.

8

I Could Do With a Break From Chemotherapy

For a lucky few, attending a chemotherapy session is almost an incidental event. They continue to work full-time, play bowls, go surfing and do many of the things they enjoy. But it would be fair to say that for most it is a more gruelling undertaking, physically and emotionally, and you should give yourself credit for enduring it.

If you're struggling, you might find your symptoms – those resulting from side effects of the therapy, such as nausea, vomiting, infections, anaemia as well as others – are treatable, or that your chemotherapy treatment can be adjusted, to make the experience more tolerable. There may well be options within your treatment to allow for a better quality of life.

Jimmy, a postman having many consecutive weeks of chemotherapy for bowel cancer, suddenly announced he could take no more after ten weeks of struggling through diarrhoea. When questioned in detail, he revealed he had been embarrassed to appear weak as he assumed that everybody suffered similarly. When I suggested we reduce the chemotherapy dose by a fraction, he said gloomily, 'I might as well not have it then.' But on hearing that the individual dose is not fixed, but rather, always needs to be adjusted according to a person's tolerance, and that a reduced dose would still be effective, he felt reassured to continue and finished the prescribed course. Six years later, Jimmy remains well and is glad he persevered.

Another suffering patient once said, 'It's rough but it's not like you can do anything. It's my cross to bear.' To the contrary, I could and did do something about her pain, which in fact was not a direct effect of chemotherapy. A single session of radiotherapy and adjustment of her morphine dose was enough to return her to her beloved garden. Before assuming that symptoms are untreatable, or that they are all side effects from chemotherapy, it is important to discuss what you're experiencing with your oncologist and look for ways to mitigate symptoms.

Hopefully you have been communicating with your oncologist all the while, but when the side effects are truly intolerable, it is definitely time to have a chat. I recommend writing down your key thoughts. Record your worst symptoms or concerns. Questions might include: How do you think this treatment is helping me? Is there an alternative? What would happen if I took a break? What would happen if I stopped treatment altogether?

I appreciate that you might think these questions are too direct. You might even fear that your doctor could be offended by you questioning or rejecting his/her treatment, or, let's face it, you might not want to know the answer. But don't overly concern yourself with being perceived as ungrateful – asked politely, these questions demonstrate your engagement in your illness and your absolute right to think over them and seek answers. Your oncologist will probably welcome the opportunity to discuss things candidly. If you are fearful about finding out bad news, limit your questions, starting with the ones you are least afraid to ask. Tell your oncologist that you want to explore your questions slowly, at your own pace. You may be surprised or relieved at the answers.

To have the confidence to ask questions, assess your reaction to treatments and make decisions about what might be best for you, you need a level head. Although it is common to start the process with anxiety and panic, and to feel that the tumult will never disappear, I can assure you that you will enter a phase where the initial shock is replaced by an acceptance, if not of the diagnosis itself, at least of the measures one needs to tackle it. It will take a few sessions, an interaction here and there with other patients, and the opportunity to get to know your medical team before you have your first chance to reflect on your situation and let things sink in.

One patient said, 'I went through four cycles of chemotherapy. There were so many setbacks that what was supposed to take three months took five. It was only when I was at the desk one day and my colleague made a casual comment about how tough it had been for me, that I thought to myself, *She's right, I have felt shocking the whole time.* Up to that point, I had never contemplated this, preferring to muddle my way through things.'

Another patient said,'I used to meet this patient in the chemo unit whose disease course was uncannily like mine. We both had incurable ovarian cancer. One day when she didn't show up, I fearfully asked my nurse what had happened. She smiled and said that the patient had decided to take a break from chemo and go on holiday. I couldn't believe my ears. "You can do that?" I exclaimed. The nurse told me that I needed to discuss it with my oncologist, but I felt such a surge of hope that day just knowing that it was possible. Until then I had never let myself think of coming off chemo although I was often tempted.' This patient and her husband discussed the idea with their oncologist at her next visit and came up with a similar plan. Her husband was clearly delighted by the unexpected break, their first in two years.

In fact, it is not uncommon for so-called chemo holidays to be both possible and beneficial, and there is a variety of reasons that might support the decision to take a break. The first thing to be considered, though, is the intent of your treatment. As I have mentioned, some types of chemotherapy and radiotherapy are delivered with the intent to cure – to kill the cancer – and these treatments may well have a window of opportunity when they are best deemed effective and which will more likely need to be completed to schedule. A break during such treatment is harder to accommodate unless there is a serious problem with continuing, such as low blood counts and infections, or an unforeseen complication such as a heart attack or bleeding, which make it unsafe to proceed. If a break for these reasons is short, perhaps one or two weeks, the rest of the therapy might then continue as planned.

Generally, curative intent means that you may have limited ability to take time off but your treatment can be modified. In many advanced forms of cancer, however, treatment is palliative, as discussed, where curing the cancer is no longer an option. The aim is to manage the cancer to stop it getting worse or to make symptoms less acute. Palliative chemotherapy therefore does not have the same defined end point – it can be continued for as long as you benefit, making it less clear to work out how much is enough. In such cases, your own insights are extremely valuable, because ultimately it should be your decision every single time to go ahead with chemotherapy. Many patients simply don't realize that there is scope for considering a break from treatment, so I hope you find the knowledge empowering.

What might be the benefits of a chemo holiday? Well, it might be best to have a break because of problems caused by the treatment. This commonly happens when you have run into serious toxicities and the emphasis is on getting you better before discussing future options. What you commonly hear is 'We'll see how you go' or 'Have a break for now and we will discuss things when you return'. Your tired body may benefit just from forgoing the exhausting travel that constant therapy requires. Then, if you recover well, you might resume the same treatment at a different dose, or possibly another type of treatment with a different side-effect profile. Sometimes the same therapy may be continued but the break means the total duration of chemotherapy might be extended.

Many patients who have been on the chemotherapy merry-go-round for months or years also find a break a welcome change to be able to reflect on what the chemotherapy has achieved so far and consider again their hopes for the future. A break from the chemotherapy unit and the 'language' of cancer can allow people to think about the other missing things from their life. Some patients determine that they don't want to spend the remainder of their life attending chemotherapy and they find the insight so revealing and refreshing that they request an extended break. They go on to enjoy good quality of life and are, in fact, pleasantly surprised by how stopping chemotherapy has made them feel better rather than worse. Other patients realize that a short break has renewed their motivation for chemotherapy and confirmed to them that it actually was making them feel better, and they return to it with fresh determination.

Some people might find stopping treatment, even temporarily, a daunting prospect in itself. Patients can worry that they are committing a fatal mistake by missing even a single session of chemotherapy, let alone deliberately foregoing it. This anxiety stems from a misunderstanding about chemotherapy. I find that many patients imagine there is a rigid protocol of treatment, where a doctor can prescribe a particular mix of chemotherapy drugs, for a fixed number of cycles, over a fixed period of time, and know for sure that it will achieve the desired result.

A common observation of patients is: 'I used to be puzzled when oncologists said they were not sure what they would do next and it depended on my situation. It took me a long time to understand what they meant.' Cancer treatment, like the treatment of many conditions, is an inexact science. Future treatment is guided by many moving pieces, some to do with you and others with advances in treatment. So if you are struggling, realizing that your treatment is not necessarily set in stone, this can be reassuring because it means you might well be able to take an occasional break without somehow reversing any progress that you have made. Oncologists know it well, but many patients describe this understanding as an important milestone in their journey.

Therefore, a discussion with your oncologist about taking a break from treatment might be about allowing you to spend some time doing something the therapy prevented, assessing how you feel about the ongoing treatment, and to prevent a dramatic decline in health. The important thing is not to feel trapped by your circumstances – to not feel that the doctors' expert opinions are the only ones that matter. You are a better expert on how you feel.

'I hate chemotherapy but my oncologist doesn't want to know about it. He dismisses my feelings saying I am lucky to be alive,' one disheartened patient confessed. While sometimes patients may feel as if their oncologist does not give them a choice and insists on treatment, the final decision always rests with you. Your oncologist might indeed say that chemotherapy is doing you good but you are entitled to think differently, especially if you are the one taking into account the subjective feelings around chemotherapy, such as how it affects you and your loved ones emotionally and how much you dread the experience.

'I have been giving her hints about being tired but my oncologist doesn't say anything,' says another patient. Sometimes, if you seem ambivalent about stopping chemotherapy your oncologist may not lead you there. She may be trying to protect your sentiments by letting you arrive at the decision to postpone treatment yourself, as she might not want you to feel unduly influenced to do so. The bottom line is that no one should have month upon month of chemotherapy with regrets. If you wish to take a break from chemotherapy, I encourage you to think about some things. Is chemotherapy making you feel better and enabling you to do some enjoyable things? Many chemotherapy regimens do just that and it's worth continuing them. But perhaps the answer was yes at an earlier time but lately has become no. Does the recovery period take longer than the first few days? A surprising number of patients go from chemotherapy to their bed to chemotherapy again. No wonder they and their carers question what good it is doing. Ask yourself what you are hoping to achieve from chemotherapy. Are you waiting to take a family holiday once you feel better? In that case, how much better would you need to feel before you went and do you think this is possible the way things are going? Would you regret not having achieved something if you were to suddenly fall too ill? Are you the kind of person who would fret if you were *not* on treatment, or would you make the most of your freedom? Talk over some of these things with someone you trust to help you review your motivation.

The availability of the riches of modern treatments means that it is not difficult for oncologists to keep prescribing different kinds of chemotherapy, sometimes only with the faintest of therapeutic benefit. This is because no doctor wants to rob the patient of hope, and because it can be uncomfortable for some doctors to discuss their limitations in treating disease. Patients look upon their oncologist as their salvation and many patients are never ready to hear that there is no other useful chemotherapy. 'I really think that she should be receiving supportive care only, but she can't bear the thought of stopping chemotherapy and I feel stuck, so I keep giving her the least toxic drug I can think of,' a colleague confided. I know that I have personally been in this unenviable situation too. You can see how patients and doctors unwittingly become tangled in a web, where neither clearly sees the benefit of continuing treatment but each hesitates to articulate it. But if you are a patient with a limited lifespan, you are right to feel an additional urgency to do what is best for you.

Do not hesitate in asking your doctor to be frank with you about the true benefits of continued treatment. For some doctors, having the patient ask is the ideal prompt for them to express views that they might otherwise find hard. You may be surprised at what you learn, either by the strong gains your doctor expects you to make, or the marginal benefit of many treatments. This knowledge may be all you need to take decisions that were otherwise hard for you.

Occasionally, patients report reluctance on the part of their oncologist to take them seriously when they wish to discuss treatment cessation, because the doctor feels this is a risky or foolish decision. 'My oncologist told my wife that the worst thing I could do was stop treatment, but he doesn't see the extent to which treatment disrupts my whole life. And I am quite prepared to live a little less in return for being able to go back to the farm, which my grandparents started. Having chemotherapy makes that impossible.' This is an observation from another patient. Sometimes an oncologist may not know you well or may not have spent enough time exploring what matters most to you. Remember that while medical decisions are based largely on evident facts, your emotional well-being matters too, and you and your family are a far better judge of the latter.

Sometimes, more vexatious than discussing a break in treatment with a reluctant oncologist is the task of dealing with loved ones who want you to continue cancer treatment even in the face of unbearable side effects. Usually the encouragement is founded on goodwill, expressed as anxiety over your welfare. Naturally, you should not dismiss their well-meant concerns. Instead, provide a gentle explanation of how the treatment makes you feel and why you have decided it is not in your best interest. Relatives and loved ones need reassurance that holistic care will not be abandoned in the process. Once they understand your situation and are themselves reassured that this is in your best interest, they will want to support you in your goals. Seeing you happier will help them and remind them of your right to choose treatment. So never continue potentially toxic measures merely for the sake of others.

Ultimately, it is up to you to declare a break from treatment or perhaps even stop it altogether, as explored in the next chapter. Before making this decision, arm yourself with objective facts via doctors and nurses, but do not ignore your own instincts, which are often the best guide to the future.

Key Points

- If you are thinking about having a break from chemotherapy, mention it to your oncologist and discuss your reasons openly.
- Specifically request your oncologist's opinion about the utility of the ongoing chemotherapy.
- Ignoring signs of chemotherapy toxicity and continuing treatment can be hazardous and even fatal. A break can make a significant difference to your well-being.
- Guilt, doubt and worry are common feelings when stopping chemotherapy but focusing on your goals will see you through.

9

When to Stop Treatment

One of the most moving occasions for me in recent times was when a dear patient with bowel cancer came in to discuss his progress. He had first been diagnosed with cancer nearly ten years ago, at which time he underwent a successful operation. He faithfully attended every follow-up, estimating that he kept close to fifty different types of appointments in the following five years. Given the all-clear, he spent the next two years living overseas with his son and grandchildren. On his return, he became unwell, initially attributing his symptoms to traveller's diarrhoea. But eventually he had some tests that showed his cancer had returned.

I had looked after him for the three years since the recurrence was diagnosed. He was initially agreeable to chemotherapy and was heartened by the results that showed impressive tumour shrinkage. An otherwise fit and robust man, he found it relatively easy to withstand the toxicities I had warned him about. He would come in each fortnight for chemotherapy, taking that day off work and returning to his office fairly quickly. Whenever he came across sicker patients in the surrounding chemotherapy chairs, he would never fail to observe how grateful he was to feel well. He joked from time to time that perhaps I wasn't giving him the 'real stuff' but he was genuinely buoyed by the fact that successive scans showed his tumour to be under good control. And it was because of this very fact that I recommended he stay on so-called maintenance chemotherapy. Oncologists have found that in certain cases keeping a patient on some form of continuous chemotherapy keeps them well longer than if chemotherapy is stopped after the traditional course. This is a relatively recent approach, only valuable in some cancers, and then only for patients who are well enough to withstand the inevitable side effects. Since my patient was tolerating chemotherapy well and continued to work and socialize, he fell in with my plan.

For years, this patient was a constant visitor to the chemotherapy unit. He became used to celebrating Easter, Christmas and other holidays with nurses, doctors and medical students. He was what we called a 'professional patient', readily offering himself as a case study for oncology trainees. We used to joke that we couldn't afford to lose him.

Four months ago, for the first time ever, he complained that he didn't feel well. His appetite was failing and instead of spending the first evening recovering from chemotherapy, he was now taking three or four days to do so. Still, he felt that his overall quality of life after those first few days of recovery was very good. Scans showed that his disease had grown slightly and we changed drugs. Very quickly his symptoms improved and he was back to the familiar cycle of a day or two of recovery followed by a good interim period. The travel back and forth had become a part of his life and he felt that as long as he had something to look forward to he would continue chemotherapy.

Two months ago, he again complained that he was unwell. His appetite was poor and his energy was fading. Scans showed his tumour had grown a little more. I gave him a complete break from treatment for a few weeks, from which he emerged feeling improved enough to cautiously try a different chemotherapy I proposed. I made small changes like reducing the dose and giving him more time off between treatments, which allowed him to give things another chance.

Recently he returned to tell me this: 'Doctor, I've lost five kilograms in the last two weeks and I'm not eating more than one meal a day. I've lost weight before, but you know what's different this time? I just can't be bothered doing anything. I'm tired and most days I just don't feel enthusiastic about getting out of bed. I've never been like this before.'

This was a clear departure from all his previous reports, where he had identified discrete and manageable problems like loss of weight or episodes of diarrhoea but never a total lack of enthusiasm to pursue treatment. In fact, while on previous occasions he had seemed keen to find ways of combating his problems, this time his tone was different. I gently asked if he was depressed. Shaking his head he replied that, on the contrary, he felt good that he had enjoyed a relatively uneventful few years despite having metastatic cancer. He asked and I told him honestly that I had not expected him to fare as well as he had. He touched on future treatment and I told him that he had exhausted most of the standard therapies, but if he still wanted to pursue treatment, there were one or two things we could give a try, although I didn't feel he was robust enough to enter a clinical trial.

'I don't expect further chemo to help me feel better, doctor,' he surmised, quite rightly.

'Unfortunately, I think you are right, but I will fit in with your wishes if you want to try something.'

'The way I've deteriorated lately,' he said, 'I feel I only have a short time left. And I would really like to slow down the pace of things, especially the trips in and out of chemo. That's the thing that I'm really over. The travel tires me almost as much as the treatment.'

I listened sympathetically and felt gratified by how well he had summarized his own situation. He had thought about the course of his illness, compared how he used to feel to how he felt now, and decided that he had had enough. He was consciously deciding to say no to further chemotherapy, which would not prolong his life but would lessen his enjoyment of the days he had left.

'I am sorry that it has come to this,' I said, upset that my best efforts had not made a bigger difference.

'Doctor, don't be sorry,' he smiled. 'I really have lived a good life and I'm ready to take it easy.'

When we said goodbye I felt sad marking the end of a good phase of his life but I was also relieved that he had made a clear decision to forgo further treatment in favour of quality of life.

It left me wishing that more patients could decide as neatly in their favour as he had and I want to spend some time discussing the matter with you.

I always listen extra carefully when a patient even hints about stopping chemotherapy. Instead of asking why, I ask them to tell me more to give them a chance to better articulate their thoughts. And the reasons are varied. Whether you are having chemotherapy for early or advanced cancer, if you are struggling and not really sure that you can get through the course, I would like you to heed some of the messages below.

Often, patients battle intolerable side effects, in which case a careful dissection of the symptoms might fix the problem. When a doctor or a nurse takes a thorough history, chemotherapy treatments can be adjusted and many side effects – such as nausea, vomiting, infections and anaemia – are treatable and, if not eradicable, can at least be alleviated to allow a better quality of life. With modern supports, many patients go through treatment with few side effects or those that are manageable. As I have mentioned previously, for a lucky few, attending a chemotherapy session is almost an incidental event, it fits in amongst other activities, but it would be fair to say that for most it is not.

In many advanced forms of cancer, treatment is palliative and not intended to improve survival. In this situation, symptom control itself is a very good aim, but if chemotherapy improves neither survival nor troublesome symptoms, it's well worth questioning its role.

But what do you do in those circumstances when despite meticulous management of side effects and complications, you struggle during chemotherapy? The struggle may be physical or emotional. I meet many patients who will not hear of having a break or stopping the very treatment that is making them ill. A common explanation is because they feel that in doing so they will fail themselves and their loved ones, that they will be giving up, but I think this is the very reason it's crucial to question the importance of chemotherapy in the bigger scheme of things.

'As long as I keep coming back for more, there is hope. If I stop chemo, I'll just be waiting to die.' This is how a seventy-seven-year-old woman described her inability to say no to chemotherapy that had landed her in hospital for the third time in a month.

Another patient's view: 'If I was single, nothing would have made me go through this. But I feel as if my wife is expecting me to pull through. I don't want her to think that I gave up.'

Both of these patients had progressive cancer. First, they were troubled by the disease itself, which was causing fatigue and shortness of breath. Then their symptoms were exacerbated by chemotherapy. However, not wanting to let down the people who were supporting them through their diagnosis, they were loath to stop treatment. It took some frank conversations to acknowledge that their illness had reached a point where no further chemotherapy would help, and moreover there was undeniable evidence that they felt weaker and worse after every cycle. In other words, their quality of life was getting poorer. More importantly, they needed to understand that the relatives they loved so much didn't want to see them suffer. We concurred that it was better for everyone to be open about the trajectory of their disease and co-opt their family into making plans for the future. Both patients stopped chemotherapy and enjoyed some good times. One patient later observed, 'Looking back, I just wish I had done this earlier. The last few weeks have been peaceful. I'm weak but feel better in my mind, if that makes sense. I think it's because I am doing very small, enjoyable things that I couldn't when I was on chemo.' The other patient's family took her to the beach after a long time; she remarked that it had been one of her most memorable experiences that year.

The question of whether or not to continue treatment becomes more pertinent when patients keep receiving chemotherapy treatments, one after the other, because nothing works for long enough. It is in this setting that you might feel tired, dispirited and vulnerable, as if you are caught in a vicious circle. 'I hate having chemotherapy but suspect I will be worse for not having it,' a long-suffering patient said. 'I just wish I had the courage to say no.'

In a few words she had summarized what I imagine many of her fellow patients silently think. Although you might understand the theory behind being fully informed about the risks and benefits of chemotherapy treatment, the reality is that you only discover what treatment entails when you start it. Part of the anxiety some people experience comes from a misconception about the role of therapy – they think that a certain number of sessions will cure the cancer, but discover to their dismay that for them the treatment will be ongoing, potentially lifelong and the best possible outcome is controlled disease rather than a cure. It is hard to predict how one might feel about being confronted with cancer. You might well have a vague plan about what you would do if your house burned down or if you became stuck without money on an overseas trip, but thinking about our own mortality is anathema. When we hear about people with cancer, we never think it could be us, even though the statistics say that by the time we reach eighty-five, one in two of us will be diagnosed with the disease. Even when an oncologist says that the chance of developing a particular complication from chemotherapy is 40 per cent, we automatically assume that we will figure in the other 60 per cent. It is human nature to allocate ourselves good odds. It is also natural in the initial panic of the diagnosis to want whatever is offered without dwelling excessively on the consequences, which might actually be useful if being consumed by anxiety paralyses you and prevents you from making decisions.

'When I was first diagnosed with breast cancer, I just did a double take. People my age were attending mothers' group and baking cupcakes. When the oncologist talked to me about chemo, I remember feeling it was such a waste of time to be even discussing these things. Of course, I wanted everything I could have and even a minute's delay seemed like an eternity. I remember feeling so overwhelmed that I said yes to everything. I can't say I understood all of it, but at that point I was so vulnerable that I was willing to put my trust in anyone who gave me any kind of hope. I went from being a competent executive to a mass of nerves.'

Does this frank admission sound familiar? But as your initial anxieties settle and side effects become pronounced, it is crucial to wonder if it's best to stop chemotherapy early despite initial recommendations. It's vital to understand that the number of cycles of chemotherapy you should have is a recommendation, not a mantra. Things may unfold during treatment that cannot be predicted by doctor or patient. It is understandable that many patients take comfort from having a clear plan of action in place – it can help to know there is an end in sight. But many factors can change in the course of treatment – including your cancer's progress, your reaction to side effects, the mental toll of treatment, and more – and it may be best to alter or even abandon the original plan. The ability to accommodate change is key to a smooth medical experience.

Robyn, a fifty-five-year-old patient, said: 'The oncologist recommended six cycles of chemotherapy. I got really sick halfway but managed to pull through the fourth. The fifth one landed me in hospital and I was too weak to stand up, let alone have the final cycle. I needed a month of rehab and felt bad that I bailed out early, but it really wasn't in my hands.'

Sri, a thirty-eight-year-old father of three, was undergoing preoperative chemotherapy to shrink his cancer before surgery when he suffered a serious reaction. He was rushed to the operating theatre where a large part of his bowel had to be removed. He was classified at extremely high risk of recurrence and every oncologist ideally recommended further chemotherapy. However, the combination of the cancer and a major operation had resulted in severe deconditioning. It took him a year to walk without the aid of a frame and recover his stamina in other ways, and chemotherapy was simply not an option.

Everyone was resigned to the fact that Sri's disease would return aggressively but many years later he remains well. Human biology is not predictable. It is impossible to know exactly how much chemotherapy an individual needs to get the best results, but we do know that the primary benefit of chemotherapy is apparent in the first few cycles. In Robyn's case, I reassured her that completing five out of six planned cycles was an excellent result, and in fact, braving the sixth cycle may have been disastrous. I advised Sri that the most important thing for him was to restore strength and feel well.

Sticking to the original plan in the face of serious problems can be catastrophic. Unfortunately, many oncologists can recall a struggling patient who has made light of the one or two more cycles of chemotherapy remaining in their treatment plan and insisted on finishing them because 'it's good to get it over with', but has subsequently ended up seriously ill, or even sometimes died as a result of overwhelming toxicity.

I can recall three or four patients who would probably have survived had they stopped their chemotherapy when they recognized that they were not coping. Instead, they were afraid that if they stopped they would be forced to return to chemotherapy later, or worse, that their disease would return as a result of incomplete treatment. Chemotherapy is not like antibiotics where failure to complete a course can render the drug inefficacious. But as a result of such misconceptions, these patients exposed themselves to unnecessary side effects and lost their life.

You might wonder in these cases why the oncologists didn't intervene since it is a doctor's obligation to keep a patient from harm. Unfortunately, many patients don't reveal the true extent of their symptoms and others insist on carrying on with treatment despite how they feel, in which case the doctor often respects their autonomy. It is another lesson in the importance of maintaining clear and open communication with your doctors.

Some of these patients had had their disease surgically removed and they were receiving treatment to reduce the chances of recurrence and hence to prolong life. One less cycle would likely have achieved just as good a result, but they didn't understand us and insisted on pressing on with the next cycle, which proved fatal. I must emphasize that death is a rare direct outcome of chemotherapy, but it is not uncommon to become unwell and even require hospitalization during treatment. If you are tolerating your treatment well, you should by all means go ahead with it because you will enjoy its benefits. But if you are struggling to manage, it's important that you acknowledge this and stop to consider your options.

The message I try to give all my patients is that chemotherapy is not a binding contract – how much, how often and how long depends entirely on the individual. I would caution you against making comparisons with other patients, even those who seem to have exactly the same disease and are receiving exactly the same treatment, because no matter what the superficial similarities, no two people have exactly the same set of circumstances.

It is a sign of the trust patients place in their oncologist that they often ask, 'What would you do if you were I?' Oncologists choose to answer this in different ways. If I know the patient and her motivations well and have witnessed the mounting side effects, I don't hesitate to say, 'If I were you, I would stop and see how I feel.' I may even say, 'I think this chemotherapy isn't doing you any favours – I would stop.' I am especially comfortable saying this when I sense that my patient has already reached this decision but is seeking my approval.

But I have colleagues who adopt a different approach, by providing the facts without weighing in on the final decision. It is not that they care less about their patients, but it is only a question of style. This is a matter of considerable debate in the medical community: What is the right balance between providing direction and encouraging patient autonomy? The answer seems to be, 'It depends on the doctor and the patient,' once again pointing to the importance of establishing a comfortable relationship with your oncologist.

Faced with a life-threatening illness, it is easy to let other people make important decisions about your health. But even if you have always relied on your doctor, your children, spouse or other people for advice, when it comes to complex things such as cancer treatment, you must be prepared to shoulder some degree of responsibility. If you have played an active role in electing whether or not to have treatment, whether to take a break or stop, and all the other decisions along the way, you will feel in control even when things don't go according to plan. Patients who passively accept whatever is recommended can feel even more powerless as they become unwell, regretting their lack of earlier involvement. If you feel that you don't understand the first thing about cancer or chemotherapy, you're probably selling yourself short because no one understands your well-being better than you. Making decisions about your chemotherapy treatment isn't easy but keeping in mind some of the considerations raised in this chapter will help.

Key Points

- If side effects are outweighing the purported benefit of treatment and your oncologist has tried to address the side effects, it may be time to stop chemotherapy.
- Stopping chemotherapy is a difficult decision even when you know it's right for you. Allow yourself time and consideration.
- Asking for honest information about the value of chemotherapy sometimes means discovering disappointing news, but you can control the amount of information you want to receive.
- Being honest with yourself and with your oncologist goes a long way towards protecting your welfare.

10

I'm Off Chemotherapy – What Now?

If you have decided to stop chemotherapy or to take a short break from it, or your oncologist has advised that you have had enough for now, it is likely that your initial relief has been replaced by trepidation about what happens next.

While on chemotherapy, you are surrounded by the 'machinery' of hospital – there are frequent tests and scans, and doctors and nurses are always hovering around. It's an odd privilege – one that you wish you didn't have – but people generally treat you with extra care when you're a chemo patient. The pathology people know you by sight because of the countless blood tests you have had and your local doctor and the emergency department fit you in as quickly as possible when you call in. The many regular appointments and odd unscheduled visits might cause logistical headaches but they are also faintly reassuring, because you feel in touch with and supported by the system. Many patients tell me that just seeing their doctors or nurses reassures them that if anything were wrong it would be picked up on. Oncology nurses seem particularly good at listening to patients, sensing their unspoken anxieties, and advocating for their needs via busy doctors. 'I always say that I am too afraid to bother my oncologist but I love the way my nurse steps up for me. I feel better having her on my side,' a neighbour told me. I knew what she meant.

But now that you are off chemotherapy, there are a number of valuable ways in which you can prepare for the future, which I'll outline here and go into in further detail in coming chapters. As an example, you can seek out a good GP, enquire about social services and link in with palliative care.

Stopping chemotherapy usually leads to a reduction in doctors' appointments, which can cause anxiety. Some patients worry about the sudden drop in the number of tests or the fact that no one is checking on them regularly. But the truth is that if you're not receiving chemotherapy, or other drugs whose side effects need to be monitored closely, you don't need to be seen by a doctor or nurse as frequently as you became accustomed to. An exception might be palliative-care support, the nature and frequency of which varies according to need.

A break from intensive cancer therapy is a good opportunity to reconnect with your primary-care physician. You are likely to have seen less of her as your chemotherapy treatment has taken precedence over any other medical assistance you may have been receiving, especially if your other conditions are stable. Also, some of your medications –such as for blood pressure, ulcer or sleeping problems – might have been renewed by your oncologist during your cancer treatment, rather than requiring visits to another physician. (It's worth noting that while this arrangement is convenient in the short term, oncologists are not always well placed to manage non-cancer concerns. Some oncologists make it a policy to not renew other prescriptions because they don't monitor your non-cancer conditions closely, in which case staying in touch with your primary-care physician during cancer treatment might be important.)

Having an accessible physician who is aware of your illness helps. Regrettably, the communication between oncologists and other doctors is not always as up to date as one would like. Sometimes the doctor who detected your cancer, or referred you to the oncologist, is not the same as your regular physician. Within your first few visits to your oncologist you should ensure that they are writing to the correct physician, especially if you have seen several in the past. It's okay, and in fact, important to check that your oncologist has sent some written communication to your primary-care physician to assist in your management, and if not, request that they do.

Some patients report that their doctors don't want to have anything to do with their cancer and automatically send them back to the oncologist with any questions. In one such case, when I called my patient's doctor and explained how some tests done at her office could help with the patient's management, the doctor was happy to recall the patient and organize the tests. The primary-care doctor then explained that she often saw hospitals duplicating any tests she had done. I understood her desire to avoid waste, but in this instance, early communication between us allowed the patient to avoid a long wait in the emergency department.

Primary-care doctors are an essential partner for both oncologist and patient and it helps everyone when they are kept abreast of your condition. Imagine if you walked in to see your doctor weeks or months after stopping chemotherapy due to severe toxicity, and he had no idea of what had been happening to you in the past few months. Many doctors feel resigned to the poor communication from specialists but others become annoyed, especially when they feel hindered in looking after someone properly. In fact, it might be a lack of information that leads a doctor to decide against becoming involved in the management of a patient's cancer.

Cancer therapies are becoming increasingly complex and sophisticated and if your doctor doesn't seem as involved in your care as you would like, remember that he or she is most likely being cautious around an unfamiliar area of expertise. It's important to tell your oncologist if your doctor is reluctant to help with your care, because the situation might be addressed by a letter or call from the oncologist to outline some common areas where you may need help. If you feel that your doctor frequently declines to deal with your cancer-related problems, you may want to think about finding a substitute. With the exception of highly specific chemotherapy-related side effects that need expert management, a primary-care doctor can capably manage almost all other common concerns. It can also be much more convenient and less anxiety-provoking to visit a physician you have known for years. I'm always humbled and secretly pleased when a patient tells me that he will discuss my recommendations with the usual physician before agreeing to anything. Patients rightly place a lot of faith in their physician – they are a source of good counsel in difficult times.

Reducing or taking a break from your cancer treatment can lead to fears that it will eventually lead to receiving no care at all. Many patients have developed a close relationship with their oncologist and rely heavily on their advice. Some refuse to let anyone draw blood other than the one nurse whom they trust. The flip side of this kind of devoted care is that it has been necessitated by a lot of time spent in an environment that has grown familiar. Patients can be thrown when they see a different oncologist, even if the advice is the same. Try to be aware that you may feel nervous when the involvement of the medical team you have come to know well diminishes.

If you are having a short or complete break from chemotherapy you can make the transition smoother by clarifying a few things upfront. Ask your oncologist how often you need to see her now that you are not on active chemotherapy. If you feel uncomfortable with the reduced frequency of check-ups, try to explain why. Is it because you don't have a regular doctor? Are you nervous that your doctor can't manage your problems? Do you simply find the visits to your oncologist more reassuring? By sharing such concerns, you are helping your oncologist come up with a plan that best suits your needs. For example, your oncologist might schedule the initial few reviews a little closer together, to temper the rate of change. In my experience, as patients feel more comfortable, they request to be seen less because they come to recognize the inconvenience of the travelling and waiting. 'Much as I like to chat with you, I'm thrilled when you say I don't need to come for another six months!' he smiled.

While some patients are relieved at requiring fewer treks to the oncologist for blood tests and scans, others feel anxious because they think no one really knows how they are doing now. This worry can be exacerbated by well-meaning relatives who dutifully ask when the next tests are due, what they show and what the oncologist thinks.

But what you should know is that the most important indicator of how you are doing is in fact how you feel and what you are able to do. If you can still mow the lawns or step out to enjoy a walk around the shops, if you can relish your favourite meal or feel enthused about going to your favourite cafe, your enjoyment of these things is an indicator that you are doing okay. However, if you are too tired to get out of your pyjamas, can't contemplate entertaining guests, can't be bothered to eat or drink as you used to, and mostly feel like resting in bed, you probably don't need a lot of invasive tests to determine you're not doing as well as you might. Doctors know the importance of clinical judgement, which means assessing your condition by looking at and listening to you.

There are some instances when certain tests and interventions have a role to play. An elderly patient of mine has prostate cancer for which he no longer receives chemotherapy. But we have agreed that he should have a periodic blood test to check for anaemia, in which case a transfusion restores his energy levels in the ensuing weeks. Another breast cancer patient undergoes weekly removal of fluid from her abdomen, which makes her feel less bloated. The first patient has a blood test via his usual doctor and the second presents directly to a radiology service with request slips that I have written in advance. Both patients have access to an oncology nurse and agree that the arrangement saves them time and avoids the delays associated with seeing me more frequently. So it is useful to discuss with your oncologist the value of any ongoing intervention and the best person to perform it, remembering that it doesn't have to be the oncologist. Being in tune with your symptoms, recognizing what kind of care helps you most, and occasionally questioning whether you need more or fewer tests, can help you keep a check on your worries and save you unnecessary pain. As always, take your cue from your own illness rather than from somebody else with the same cancer, as their situation may be very different to yours in ways in which you are not aware.

A key aspect of managing your transition from hospital-based care, led by specialist doctors and nurses, to that based in the community has to do with setting up the right resources. You should talk to your oncologist early about whether palliative care is appropriate for you. We will discuss in detail in a later chapter what palliative care entails, but, in brief, where they exist, community palliative care teams provide an extension of medical support in your own home. Such a team mostly involves trained nurses who liaise with your oncologist and other relevant specialists to manage a variety of symptoms. The focus is on avoiding unnecessary hospital admission, controlling symptoms and allowing them to stay in the comfort of familiar surroundings. You may also need a physiotherapist and occupational therapist to advise on aids and house modifications that can make it easier for you to be at home. Council supports for domestic cleaning and personal hygiene, meal delivery services, meditation groups and volunteer visits are some other services you might find useful. Your primary-care doctor can help you access them or in some cases, you can self-refer. Depending on how you feel, you may want to adopt or resume a hobby. If you are presently well, don't dismiss volunteer visits or meal and cleaning services; rather, keep them in mind for the future, remembering that they may have a waiting list.

A reduction in visits to the oncologist and chemo nurses, and stepping away from the busy but reassuring pace of a chemotherapy unit, naturally feels like a big change. Part of you welcomes it and is relieved but another part can fret. I would advise you not to view this change as a loss of care, but a transition in the intent of care. Welcome the opportunity to capitalize on your quality of life and good luck with it.

Key Points

- It is normal to feel anxious when you stop chemotherapy. But it does not mean stopping your care.
- Where available, explore and take advantage of a range of community supports.
- Be clear about what, if any, blood tests and scans you need, when you need them, and how the results are helpful, or not, to your follow up. Understanding this can reduce anxiety and misconception.
- Have a trusted primary-care doctor who is familiar with your management. Ensure that correspondence from your oncologist to your usual doctor is up to date.

11

Do I Need Radiotherapy?

Radiotherapy or radiation therapy refers to the use of X-rays to target cancer cells in the body. Unlike chemotherapy, which involves tablets, needles, intravenous drips and so on, radiotherapy is like having an X-ray, with treatment lasting just a few minutes. The procedure itself doesn't cause pain. However, as we will discuss, there are some side effects of radiotherapy for which you may need medication.

Radiotherapy has proven itself to be a successful and valuable component of cancer therapy. As with chemotherapy, it is an evolving field. Modern radiation oncologists have a number of tools at hand to decide how best to help you.

Delivered in single doses called fractions, radiotherapy can be used as a stand-alone treatment before, during or after chemotherapy. The intention is always to target rapidly dividing tumour cells and destroy them. Depending on the nature of your cancer and its location, radiotherapy might achieve a cure or provide good symptom relief. Some cancers are more sensitive to radiotherapy than others, and different organs tolerate different doses of radiation too. You can receive radiation in a single fraction, a few fractions or for several weeks, depending on the goal.

Radiotherapy is usually delivered like an X-ray, which means that you are positioned on a table with shields to protect uninvolved body parts, before a machine emits some rays to treat you. Sometimes you need to wear a cast or some other support to stabilize the part of your body that is being treated. You will be advised of this during your planning session, which, among other things, involves taking fresh scans of the cancer to allow the radiation scientist and doctor to position your treatment. Unlike chemotherapy, which is usually given in a day unit where there are surrounding chairs and patients, radiation is administered in an enclosed room where there is only one patient at a time. Each treatment of radiotherapy takes only a few minutes but correct positioning of the equipment requires extra time. The staff will step out when you are having the actual treatment. Some people worry that having radiotherapy makes them radioactive and hence make them unable to see or touch family members, but they need not fear. External radiotherapy – the commonest form of radiotherapy – doesn't make you radioactive and you don't need to take any special contact precautions.

Internal radiotherapy is a less common form of radiation typically used for tumours of the prostate and cervix. It differs from external radiotherapy in that a radioactive seed is implanted in the patient, which emits radiotherapy for a duration and intensity directed by the supervising doctor. Patients do become mildly radioactive during this time and should ask their doctor about precautions.

Depending on your tumour you may also come across terms such as gamma knife stereotactic surgery and stereotactic radiotherapy, intensity-modulated therapy and proton beam therapy. These advanced forms of external radiotherapy rely on more precise definition of the target area so as to kill cancer cells but preserve greater areas of normal tissue than traditional forms of treatment, which provide the maximum tolerable dose that will not harm normal tissue.

Stereotactic surgery doesn't mean having an operation – rather, it is a term used for a single treatment, or occasionally a few, of stereotactic radiotherapy. Stereotactic radiotherapy with a gamma knife is used on highly sensitive areas like the brain and involves wearing a frame that is surgically fixed to the skull so that there is no movement during treatment. It is generally associated with fewer side effects and better quality of life, as it doesn't interfere with normal tissue to the same degree as standard radiotherapy. However, it is a newer and more specialized technique that may not be widely available. It is also not suitable for tumours that are too large, multiple in number, or in certain locations best discussed with your radiation oncologist.

Intensity-modulated radiotherapy allows different parts of a tumour to receive different doses of radiation as judged appropriate by a radiation specialist. This allows the tumour to be targeted while limiting damage to surrounding tissues. Proton beam therapy is a new form of radiation that causes fewer side effects because the beams can only penetrate to a certain depth in the body, again meaning that the targeted cancer is destroyed without the X-rays reaching the surrounding normal tissue.

As technology improves, doctors are constantly looking for ways to improve administering radiotherapy to minimize its harm. The goal is to limit toxicity, which in some instances can be quite severe. Whether you receive one form or another of radiotherapy and precisely what instrument is used are determined by unique factors that are best discussed by a radiation oncologist. More important than the actual type of radiotherapy is the total dose, your ability to tolerate it and what it aims to achieve in the first place. Examples of possible aims of radiotherapy treatment include cure, stabilization of disease without cure, and symptom relief from pain, bleeding, etc.

A patient of mine recently declared, 'There's no way I'm having chemotherapy – I saw what it did to my grandma. But I will have radiotherapy because I heard from my friend that she didn't feel a thing. After all the things I've been through, I like the idea of a non-toxic treatment.' Alas, there is no such thing as a non-toxic cancer therapy and my poor patient received a rude surprise when radiotherapy to her breast resulted in a more severe than usual skin reaction, which became infected and painful. So I want to spend a little bit of time discussing the variety of side effects of radiotherapy, which, as a rule, increase with the number of fractions you receive.

Fatigue is an especially common accompaniment due to the amount of travel involved for many patients. Radiotherapy centres are not always nearby chemotherapy units, so if you are receiving combined therapy, this might mean travelling from chemo in the morning to radiotherapy in the afternoon. If you are receiving only radiotherapy and need more than one session, the sessions will be held on consecutive days, with weekends off. Five sessions of radiotherapy will mean travelling back and forth to the centre for five days of the week and having the weekend off. Some patients are recommended radiotherapy twice a day. It is really useful to have someone drive you during radiotherapy because you will be tired. An escort can also help you pass the time and ward off nervousness or boredom while you wait.

Vomiting is not very common with radiotherapy but can occur. Nausea and loss of appetite are typical side effects. The radiation oncologist will prescribe medication that you can take beforehand to combat these effects. With prolonged radiotherapy and ongoing nausea and appetite loss, you may begin to lose weight that you can ill-afford. If you find you don't feel like eating normal meals it's important to eat small meals more frequently, and to use supplements such as protein drinks between meals or as meal replacements.

Skin changes can range from dryness, flaking and a mild rash to blistering, ulceration and infections. These changes don't happen overnight and proper skin care can avoid many of the problems. You will be asked to avoid harsh soaps, perfumes and excessive sun exposure. You may also need special gels, washes, creams or dressings to protect the affected area, which will usually improve after you finish radiotherapy.

Treatment to the head and neck, oesophagus and stomach area can lead to local inflammation and difficulty swallowing. Destruction of the salivary glands in the mouth can lead to permanent difficulty with salivation, and hence, dryness of the mouth. This in turn can mean difficulty chewing food properly, mouth ulcers and dental decay. If you have pre-existing dental problems, or you are worried about these effects, your doctor may suggest seeing a dentist before treatment.

When oesophageal cancer in particular is treated with protracted courses of radiotherapy, the difficulty with swallowing can become problematic. Many patients complain of such a strong burning sensation that they refuse to eat and drink and end up in hospital with dehydration and malnutrition. Once this occurs, it is a very slow process to get patients back on their feet – it takes far longer to salvage your condition than to create it. Therefore, it's the routine practice of many radiotherapy doctors to discuss the pre-emptive placement of a feeding tube (a nasogastric tube) to allow adequate nutrition to continue during radiotherapy. The tube, inserted through the nose and down the throat, will usually remain in place for the duration of treatment, and then some more weeks while healing occurs. A nasogastric tube does not require sedation or anaesthetic to insert or remove. Most patients describe a nasogastric tube as temporarily uncomfortable or annoying but not painful. It bothers some more than others. Bear in mind that for some patients having a nasogastric tube is a 'deal breaker'. They dislike the idea of tube feeding and will not accept a course of radiotherapy that compels them to do so. Discuss this with your doctor beforehand.

Treatment to the lower abdomen is associated with nausea, vomiting, diarrhoea and urinary irritation. Skin inflammation and breakdown and minor bleeding can also occur. Despite normal organs being shielded from the X-rays, healthy structures like ovaries and testicles may be affected – their function may diminish or even cease as a result of radiotherapy. This depends on your age, the amount and site of radiotherapy and accompanying chemotherapy. Both men and women contemplating having a family should seek specialist fertility advice before cancer treatment. Fertility experts are familiar with the need for expedited counselling and assistance with fertility preservation to avoid delays in cancer treatment.

From a practical perspective, I find many patients enter chemotherapy expecting it to be gravely toxic but underestimate the side effects that radiotherapy can cause. But the situation is more nuanced these days. Many modern chemotherapies – and especially targeted therapies – do not carry the conventional, feared side effects, and radiotherapy is not always free from problems. As you can see from the descriptions above, radiotherapy can be onerous too. Radiation oncologists are good at taking patients through what to expect, but you should ask questions if you are still not sure.

A few of my radiotherapy patients come to mind when discussing what to expect. A seventy-five-year-old lady received five weeks of chemotherapy and radiotherapy for locally advanced pancreatic cancer, after being advised that the tumour was inoperable but had a small chance of being cured with combined treatment. Upon hearing about the side effects she vacillated before convincing herself to go ahead. She hated every day of treatment. Three weeks after finishing she presented with intense nausea and loss of weight. I initially reassured her that she was probably suffering the final effects of treatment, which would soon abate. However, an ultrasound of her liver showed that the cancer had spread to her liver. Her specialists concluded that it was likely that the tumour had been there all along while she was receiving treatment. She was incredulous, and later devastated, to learn that she had put herself through 'months of misery' without any benefit.

She declined all further chemotherapy for metastatic pancreatic cancer, refused to see her doctors again and died a few months later. She told me that her chief regret was receiving radiotherapy because it had particularly hampered her quality of life. She expressed the thought that if she had understood the gravity of her disease and realized that cure was unlikely she would have acted differently.

I discussed this with her radiation doctor who was also upset at the outcome. However, the doctor explained that it was clear in retrospect that the patient had frequently downplayed her symptoms, preferring a 'let's just get on with it' approach. She had been so eager to finish her treatment that she had avoided letting on too much about how poorly she was feeling, which may have led her doctors to reconsider their plan. They may have discovered the progression of her cancer sooner.

In contrast, a young patient with lung cancer benefited greatly over two years with episodic radiotherapy applied to painful bony spread to her pelvis. Successful resolution of her most troublesome symptom – the pain – helped her defer chemotherapy, and the radiotherapy itself caused no mentionable side effects because it was given in small doses. For her, radiotherapy was a very good alternative to having chemotherapy and allowed her to spend quality time with her children.

A third patient started so-called prophylactic radiotherapy to the brain after his lung cancer appeared cured. Prophylactic radiotherapy is given to a body part where doctors believe occult cancer cells are likely to aggregate in the future. The knowledge is based on experience with previous patients with the same disease. Although he had tolerated chemotherapy reasonably well he was so tired from it that the brain radiotherapy compounded his fatigue and made him very ill. He felt nauseous and giddy, found his attention span diminishing and was deteriorating by the day. He had been a robust octogenarian but now feared he would forever lose his quality of life. So, after discussion with his radiation oncologist, he decided to stop treatment. He told me that he had been made aware that the side effects would abate with time. He struggled with the notion that he was giving up on potential benefits but ultimately decided that he would rather take the chance than subject himself to radiotherapy. He also calculated that at his age, cancer was not the only risk to his life, but also his diabetes and heart disease. His radiation oncologist was very supportive and continued to monitor him regularly. The man lived a long and healthy life subsequently and died not of recurrent cancer but a heart attack. His wife felt that he had lived well in the interim years and never once regretted his decision to stop radiotherapy.

I hope you see that the point I am making is that as with any treatment, radiotherapy can help or hinder. Your response depends on a number of the factors we have discussed. As with chemo, it is vital to understand your choices and make an informed decision. Questions you should ask your radiation oncologist include the aim of treatment, its likely duration (days or weeks) and the anticipated side effects (both short- and long-term). Remember that doctors can sometimes unintentionally skim over side effects that mean a great deal to particular patients. If brain radiotherapy may cause vague memory loss or difficulty in concentrating, only you can tell how much this will affect your quality of life. The same goes for nausea, infertility, diarrhoea or other problems. Ask also if radiotherapy will be combined with chemo, causing additive toxicity. It may be pertinent to understand how much additional benefit will be gained from prolonged radiotherapy as opposed to a short course, and indeed, whether radiotherapy is essential to have, or whether observation or chemotherapy alone may suffice. Sometimes the benefit of treatment is small. It's important to appreciate this because it helps you make an informed choice as to what side effects you are willing to put up with. It also means that if you choose to stop treatment, you may not feel so bad about it.

Unfortunately, a lot of what we do in medicine (all of medicine, not just cancer) is not backed by as robust a body of evidence as we might like. Doctors also act from experience and gut instinct. This doesn't mean that our practice is completely random, but it does allow room to fine-tune treatment to every individual patient. Just because doctors have always done something one way doesn't mean that they cannot consider a different way for you. And if you don't ask, you won't ever know what is possible.

Always be honest with your doctor about your priorities, and what you are and aren't willing to accept. A good doctor–patient relationship is based on mutual understanding, not pressure to follow one prescribed path. If you have started radiotherapy but find yourself having second thoughts, bring this up with your doctor. For all you know, some problems might be easily fixed, allowing you to finish treatment as planned. Some patients report feeling silly mentioning toxicities that they were told to expect. But doctors mention potential side effects from a long list, not able to know in advance which ones will bother you the most or the least. Only you can explain this once the treatment has begun; so naturally, this is the time to adjust things. Your oncologist will usually have close contact with the radiation doctor so you can also mention your concerns to the oncologist.

Radiotherapy is a very valuable arm of cancer therapy. By ensuring that you openly communicate with your radiation doctor, you can make sure you use it to your best advantage.

Key Points

- Radiotherapy is a valuable component of cancer treatment. It is delivered in the form of rays directed at a particular part of the body affected by cancer.
- Radiotherapy is toxic, is given for short durations and usually cannot be employed repeatedly in the same area of the body.
- The decision to include radiotherapy as treatment is made by a radiation oncologist, usually in concert with an oncologist.
- Discussing the aim of radiotherapy with your radiation oncologist will help you manage expectations.

12

Why Can't I Have an Operation to Remove the Cancer?

'I don't care about anything else, but please tell me it's operable.' This retired teacher's plea is a familiar refrain when somebody discovers a new cancer diagnosis. After the initial shock, it's natural to want to know if the cancer can be cut out and removed forever.

'It is operable,' I replied, looking at the scans, 'but I'm not sure it is curable.'

'Isn't that just semantics, doctor?' he asked tiredly. 'Operable means curable, in my book.'

Most people share the misconception that cancer surgery implies a cure. They think that if a surgeon can get to their cancer it can be permanently removed and they will have a better chance of survival. So if you are told your cancer is operable, you might feel instantly relieved, although the road to recovery is often long and complicated. Alternatively, if you are told your cancer is inoperable, it can lead to intense foreboding and anxiety.

Often the question of surgery isn't as clear-cut as you might hope. 'How difficult can it be to get a yes or no answer?' one patient grumbled. 'Isn't that what surgeons do?'

I explained to the teacher that his bladder cancer indeed required an operation to avoid some foreseeable complications, but his cancer looked too widespread for the urologist to be sure that the surgery would result in a complete cure. It was likely that cells had spread beyond the bladder to involve other local organs that could not be operated on so easily. Eventually, with the aid of drawings and further discussion, he understood my point, but he learned for himself the difficulty of explaining it to his family. 'I can assure you that the average person doesn't differentiate between operability and curability,' he told me.

I want to discuss cancer surgery with you from an oncologist's viewpoint. The aim is not to explore the specifics of any particular cancer operation – which only your operating surgeon should do – but to help you understand the broader concept of the role of surgery in cancer.

In modern times, some cancers, such as those involving the breast, bowel and prostate, are diagnosed via screening tests. Sometimes cancer is incidentally detected on X-rays conducted for other reasons. An elderly lady with a broken arm needed a chest X-ray prior to surgery and the X-ray revealed a lung cancer that had never given her any symptoms. Another patient had a CT scan for abdominal pain and was incidentally found to have a kidney cancer, which was then safely removed.

If your cancer diagnosis started with the discovery of a suspicious mass, you will know that multiple other tests are subsequently performed to ensure that the mass is cancerous, localized in one area, and safe and practical to operate on. The tests are time-consuming but important. The ideal outcome in these instances is the complete removal of the cancerous tumour, ensuring the least chance of future spread.

Like chemotherapy, advances in surgical technique and the availability of newer, more sophisticated and accurate technology mean that surgery that was not previously deemed possible may now be contemplated. This decision ultimately rests in the hands of the surgeon and patient. The type and volume of surgical expertise available in a hospital are an important factor in determining operability and outcomes. It sometimes happens that what one surgeon considers inoperable another surgeon may not – different equipment, more specialized training, years of experience and ancillary support services play a role in this.

Some years ago I met a patient who had been deemed inoperable at one hospital. A large academic centre argued that this advice had been premature. The patient was disappointed by the perceived failure of the first surgeon to advise him more thoroughly and eagerly accepted an operation. The surgery went ahead but the patient spent nine weeks in intensive care and when he was finally discharged, he was too weak to walk. Also, as the original surgeon had worried, the cancer could not be safely removed and a significant portion of disease was left behind. However, chemotherapy could not be administered safely due to the patient's weakness. He later expressed regret at jumping to the conclusion that an operation was always better. 'I guess I was sold on the fact that someone thought that an aggressive approach was the best.' I advise all my patients that, like chemotherapy, no surgery, however minor, is risk-free.

If you have been declined surgery, it is worth discussing whether you should obtain a second opinion. Sometimes, another opinion can make all the difference. I know a butcher who had had an operation for throat cancer at a major cancer centre. His surgeon had warned him that one side effect of the curative surgery was a hoarse voice, but in the ensuing months he found that his voice was much worse than he'd expected. He was unable to call out his wares at the farmer's market and felt dispirited about leaving his job. His son was concerned that if his father stayed away from the shop, he would sink into depression. This fear led the family to researching their options.

One day the son told me that they had found a new operation that promised to restore his father's voice, but it was only available in another state. 'I just don't know whether this is a sham operation or something we should consider. I'm lost.' My first instinct was to recommend caution when going to an unfamiliar place to an unknown surgeon, especially when the butcher lived in a major city that offered a very high standard of cancer care. But when he insisted that the operation seemed 'genuine', I told him to talk to his own surgeon. If indeed the technology wasn't available locally, his surgeon would probably be glad to recommend going elsewhere. But if the procedure was unproven, unsafe, or simply inappropriate, there was no one better placed than the surgeon to know that.

The butcher's son paled at the thought of 'challenging' his surgeon, wanting to quietly take his dad interstate. But eventually he took my advice and was pleasantly surprised at the outcome. The first surgeon expressed sympathy at the patient's ongoing problem and agreed that the new procedure was worth a try. The two surgeons spoke, the patient flew interstate, and his voice improved so well that he was back at work within weeks. His follow-up was arranged locally with the first surgeon, reducing the need for repeated travel. This is a good example of someone who benefited from a second opinion as a result of cooperation between specialists. From time to time one hears about doctors' inflated egos inhibiting information-sharing and recommendations for more appropriate care but, in my experience, most doctors genuinely work towards the best outcomes for their patients.

While there are cancers that can be completely treated via surgery, some may be deemed technically operable – that is, surgery is possible – but other factors mean an operation may not necessarily be the best thing for the patient. So-called locally advanced diseases fall into this category. An example is locally advanced lung cancer. In this condition, lung cancer has spread to the nearby lymph glands but not distant organs such as the liver or bones. Another instance is that of locally advanced pancreatic cancer, where the proximity of the cancer to important blood vessels determines its operability. There are many other such examples but in all, patient preference plays an important role in decision making.

Here are some things I ask my patients to think about when contemplating surgery. Surgery for your cancer may be complicated and require prolonged time in an operating theatre, thus increasing the chances of anaesthetic and post-operative complications. An extended stay in hospital may be required, perhaps including time in intensive care, as well as the commonly known complications of hospitalization including infections, falls, confusion, the need for artificial feeding and hydration and so on. And, of course, the operation may be just the first step in a much longer journey of cancer therapy demanding your energy.

Sometimes, even if your cancer is potentially operable, the surgeon might advise against it because her experience suggests that the cancer is likely to be more advanced or difficult to remove than scans suggest. Patients are surprised that doctors can have this doubt despite looking at the most sophisticated scans, but even these scans have limitations. An experienced surgeon may determine that there is enough likelihood of spread and that major surgery would do more harm than good. There is no substitute for the gut instinct of an experienced surgeon.

An operation is never an isolated procedure. Even if two people have the same illness, an operation will not yield the exact same results. A frail woman with severe emphysema, requiring a portable oxygen cylinder at home, is no candidate for thoracic surgery even if a small lung cancer can be technically removed. She would not survive the operation. Such a patient is likely to be sent to an oncologist or a radiation oncologist for an opinion.

A surgeon recently advised avoiding aggressive pancreatic surgery in a man already severely malnourished and at risk of further deterioration during a prolonged hospital stay. Pancreatic surgery requires you to be very fit. Age itself does not automatically rule out having an operation but having other serious conditions can. A fifty-seven-year-old with pre-existing heart and kidney failure has a worse prospect than a fit and active seventy-year-old with no major health problems. A patient with dementia may be expected to experience complications that a normal patient would not. When contemplating surgery, the focus should not be on the procedure alone but on the complete health and fitness of the patient. Talk to your family and your primary-care doctor about what complications, physical and emotional, you might expect and how you might cope. Finally, in borderline cases, you should consider if there is a reasonable alternative to surgery. It is possible that modern chemotherapy and/or radiation therapy may deliver an equally good outcome and be the best way for you to preserve quality of life by sparing surgery.

Unfortunately, a significant number of cancers are diagnosed at a late stage, which makes surgery not possible. Although overall cancer survival rates are improving, there are still significant numbers of patients diagnosed with advanced or metastatic cancer – cancer that has spread around the body. It is also commonly referred to as Stage IV cancer. Due to well-established screening tests, only about 10 per cent of women are now diagnosed with metastatic breast cancer and just 20 per cent of patients with colon cancer have late-stage disease. But upwards of 50 per cent of patients with lung cancer and pancreatic cancer and nearly 70 per cent of women with ovarian cancer are diagnosed with an advanced stage of disease. This happens because some cancers don't cause early-warning symptoms and have no well-established screening tests.

The majority of metastatic cancer cannot yet be cured by surgery because, by definition, it has spread beyond one site. Usually, an oncologist will resort to some form of chemotherapy to tackle metastatic disease. In some instances when cancer has spread to a very limited number of sites, it may be possible for surgery to remove them all and prolong survival. Traditionally, colon cancer that had spread also to the liver was incurable. However, modern expertise allows the oncologist and surgeon to work together to remove liver metastases. But such patients are still rare – their disease needs to be of small volume and in the right geographical location. Similarly, neurosurgery can successfully remove a brain metastasis located in an accessible area. It is always gratifying to see someone recover well and carry on with his or her usual activities without losing balance or having a seizure.

If you have advanced cancer you may still require an operation to deal with a current or predicted complication, but usually your doctors will rely on other modes of therapy to treat the cancer fully. A patient of mine recently had a kidney removed via keyhole surgery because his kidney cancer kept bleeding and developing infections. The kidney was removed to allow him a better quality of life, but he still required chemotherapy to tackle the rest of his cancer. For the majority of patients with advanced cancer, surgery is futile and even detrimental as it doesn't extend survival and, in fact, may do the opposite by exposing them to complications.

I'm sure someone has helpfully told you about someone else who has the same kind of cancer who was cured by an operation. Like many people, you may be curious to know more. There is an understandable tendency for patients to compare their situation with those of other patients. Some are known to wonder whether it is their lack of connections that has led them to miss out on surgery, or inadequate expertise on the part of their doctors. Others feel dissatisfied because they were simply told that they were inoperable without any further explanation. Some insist that a patient who was in exactly the same situation received surgery while they themselves were passed over. I hope you now understand that it's usually because the two patients were not in fact comparable – there are many factors that may differ for each individual.

Many misgivings you might have can be corrected by communication. Write down your questions and share them with your doctor, oncologist and other qualified professionals you will meet. More information about the location of your disease or type of cancer may be the clarification you need. These days, there are ample opportunities for an oncologist or a patient to consult more than one surgeon if there is a question about the benefit of surgery, so don't hesitate to ask for another opinion if you are not convinced. Ask to see diagrams and other helpful resources if you need.

Generally speaking, where expertise exists, cancer surgeons will not hesitate to operate if your chances are favourable. But if surgery has little to offer, and could potentially cause further harm, it is appropriate to avoid it. Needless to say, there are also patients who, after weighing up the possible benefits and drawbacks, decline an operation. You shouldn't hesitate to do this if you have a feeling that intensive surgery isn't for you. I recently saw a patient whose daughter was concerned that his dementia was worsening as rapidly as the cancer on his ear on which the surgeon had advised a major operation. Confronted with a genuine dilemma, the family decided to avoid surgery in favour of quality of life, and they never looked back. Remember that spending some time understanding a few details of your cancer and also how your diagnosis fits in with the rest of your health and your wishes for care will avoid many unanswered questions and delayed regrets.

Key Points

- Many cancers, especially those detected at a late stage, are not curable by an operation.
- An operation does not always indicate cure. Find out what an operation will achieve for you and what other cancer treatment you will require.
- It's okay to seek a second opinion.
- Before you consent to an operation, clearly understand the implications.
- It is okay to decline surgery if what is described does not fit in with your expectations.You are the patient and your views are most important.

13

Is a Clinical Trial for Me?

'I will take anything you throw at me; put me in one of those trials, doctor.' Martin's cancer had responded well to the standard treatments for two years before he started experiencing progressive disease and a worsening of his condition. In the next several months he went through many other available therapies, but was disappointed at finding each response short-lived. He had always been fit and now, despite his cancer, could not sit idle. On days when the pain was controlled he would enjoy reading a novel or potter around in his workshop. When fatigue set in, he would spend the day on the sofa but keep his mind active by doing crosswords. So when I told him that we had exhausted all available options for treatment, he didn't feel he was quite ready to accept the news. He was reasonable and insightful, but also had a real zest for life. 'I know I can't be cured, but I will try anything out there to give me some more time.' We talked about finding a suitable clinical trial and what it might involve. Fortunately, a trial of a new drug opened a month after our conversation and I had Martin assessed for eligibility. He met the criteria and was buoyed by receiving a fresh chance. He discovered to his pleasure that he tolerated the new therapy better than any of his previous ones. His illness remained stable, and his quality of life very good, for far longer than either of us had imagined. When his cancer had spread despite being on standard therapies, he was resigned that he would deteriorate quickly. But he said that the new drug had acted as a lifesaver for him. Certainly, it was wonderful to see him looking so well and feeling hopeful again.

Cheered by Martin's experience, I encouraged another patient, Sergei, to join the same trial. He was somewhat younger but had roughly similar characteristics to Martin. When Sergei's chemotherapy failed, after a year and a half, his daughter, who was his primary carer, was keen for him to try something else. I wasn't so sure that Sergei would be interested in the trial, but I broached it with him, wanting him to be informed of all options. As I had expected, he initially declined but, nudged by his daughter, he reconsidered and decided to give the drug a try. Unfortunately, Sergei's experience was the opposite of Martin's.

From the start, Sergei hated providing multiple blood samples and the long travel and waiting time in clinic. He complained that just in the first month he experienced all of the mentioned side effects and none of the promised benefits. Yet he persisted unhappily for another few weeks. Then, just as he was about to come off trial, he suffered an allergic reaction and was admitted to hospital with a serious rash, kidney failure and delirium. He spent two weeks in hospital, coming close to death. Needless to say he stopped all treatment. Sergei told me that he regretted the time that participation in the trial had eaten up. 'If I had thought about it, I would have taken myself fishing instead.' He refused to believe that anyone on the trial had a positive experience.

The experiences of these two men have since served me as a good reminder to be discriminatory about enrolling patients on clinical trials. If you have been through all the usual therapies for your cancer, it's natural for you to wonder whether there is anything else available. You may have heard of a ground-breaking or miracle treatment popularized by the media – to the dismay of many oncologists, patients source a lot of information from sensational current affairs shows that bear little resemblance to real life.

If you have any involvement with cancer you will hear mention of a clinical trial, and indeed, you may be keeping your ears close to the ground to hear of something that might benefit you or someone you care for. At any time, there are probably hundreds and hundreds of trials taking place all over the world that are in various stages of development, but they all have one quest – how to beat cancer. A trial can do both good and harm and if you are considering entering one, it's advisable to be aware of its benefits and limitations. Although patients sign consent forms, the nature of the explanations they receive and how much is actually understood is a lively topic of debate in the medical community. Suffice it to say, the vulnerability of patients, who have failed all conventional forms of therapy and will grasp at any straw, is well recognized and doctors do their best to put safeguards in place. While emphasizing that you should thoroughly read your particular consent form, I want to spend some time telling you about the basics of a clinical trial.

A clinical trial is an experiment that tests the effectiveness of a new drug for a given disease. The drug being tested might be in a formulation such as a tablet, injection, intravenous chemotherapy or a skin patch. The growth in our understanding of cancer biology has meant an explosion in the number of clinical trials, with scientists eager to try out ideas from the laboratory on actual patients, so-called bench-to-bedside medicine. Whereas once clinical trials were limited to the largest hospitals with plentiful resources, nowadays even smaller and regional centres are participating in feasible trials. Most are so expensive to run that they are sponsored, funded or in some way supported by pharmaceutical companies, which naturally have a vested interest in the success of their product. Large pharmaceutical companies employ professional writers to write manuscripts. It's no secret that they pay key opinion leaders to speak positively about their drugs. The fortunes of a pharmaceutical company can rest on the success of a single cancer drug; so it is wise to be aware that there may be bias in the reporting of trials. Having said this, it is by means of well-conducted clinical trials that medicine moves forward, so they deserve our support.

I want to touch now on the different kinds of trials, which becomes important when you evaluate your chances of benefitting from participation. Phase I and Phase II trials are trials in their early stages. They are used to provide answers to very basic but crucial questions: Is this drug safe in humans? What is the appropriate dose of the drug? Does it have any unacceptable side effects? A Phase I trial evaluates a drug in a small number of patients, exploring the best way to deliver it and its optimal dose. A Phase II trial expands the treatment to a larger number of patients. Scientists explore whether it works while they assess its overall safety. So-called 'positive' results in these early-phase trials are liberally defined. A positive finding may mean that the small patient group did not suffer any adverse effects. Or that the level of a tumour marker, a protein secreted by tumour cells, decreased, or there were some other microscopic features of the tumour that improved.

It is important to understand that early-phase trials don't have cure as their goal – they are the baby steps that a company takes to test a hypothesis. A promising idea on paper doesn't automatically translate into a good result for patients – as a result, the vast majority of Phase I and Phase II trials, nearly 90 per cent in fact, fail to go any further. Incidentally, this is also the reason why a successful cancer product is so expensive – to recoup the cost of all the previous failed trials.

Phase III trials are conducted with hundreds or even thousands of patients, to test an experimental drug either against the current standard medication in use or a placebo (a dummy treatment with no effects), to establish whether the new drug is better, worse or equivalent to existing drugs. Phase III trials are often referred to as the 'gold standard' in trials, because a well-conducted trial gives oncologists vital, practical information about whether to use a therapy on current patients. The results, often announced amidst great fanfare at major conferences, can change patient management overnight. I will never forget emerging from a large international conference and waiting for my flight when I overheard a person, who must have been an oncologist, call his mother: 'Mum, I've just heard some great positive data on pancreatic cancer. Tell your doctor to hold off your chemo until we've talked. I don't know whether he's heard.'

I have been gratified by how the revelations of some of these large trials have genuinely helped my patients, and when I look back over just the last decade of my practice, I can see how much the landscape has changed thanks to good, informative clinical trials. But as the interpretation of trials can be subject to bias, results that seem striking on paper don't always deliver in real life.

In a clinical trial where the effect being measured is small – for example, a delay of four weeks in cancer progression, or survival extended by one month – it is possible that the result has occurred purely by chance. Also, while it is well known that scientific publications are full of reports of positive trials (meaning trials that show a benefit, however small), a lot of negative trials that reveal that a new treatment is no better than the existing one remain unpublished, even though they can be just as informative for the clinician.

'Doctor, my friend's niece works day and night in a cancer research lab – how can you tell me there is nothing new for my cancer? Where does all the research go?' This patient of mine was asking a very good question. Despite the proliferation of clinical trials it is actually difficult to identify truly well-conducted and sufficiently large trials from which to draw meaningful conclusions. Even then, clinical trials simply cannot match the eventual biological and genetic diversity of the patients in the community who will be taking the drug, which is why a drug that seems to do well in a controlled environment with a relatively small group of patients doesn't always perform as well on the wider population. Patients who participate in a trial are carefully selected and closely monitored. They tend to be young and robust, nurses remind them to take their pills, they are subjected to frequent tests that monitor small changes, and side effects they experience are quickly reined in. As any oncologist will tell you, these conditions don't reflect 'real-life' patients, who are usually elderly, may not like taking prescribed medication, and battle against additional chronic and complex conditions.

I draw your attention to all of this not to take away any hope that clinical trials might benefit you, but to help you assess trials in a clearer light. Early-phase clinical trial drugs – those Phase I and Phase II drugs in the early stages of being tested – are many years away from entering the market, and regrettably, a significant majority will be found to be ineffective despite initial promising results. Late-phase trial drugs can also take many years to be approved, even if their potential benefits are borne out by other trials. Regulatory authorities in different countries have varying rules about whether a drug should be approved, depending on cost, perceived benefit and other considerations. For example, UK and Australian patients may find that cancer therapies available in the United States are not funded in their countries. This is usually because their government-funded health care system may have concluded that the drug is not cost-effective or that a reasonable alternative exists. Sometimes governments wait to negotiate a better price with a pharmaceutical company.

We all know that serendipity plays a part in science and medical researchers stumble upon unexpected discoveries that go on to help large numbers of patients. But if you participate in an early-phase trial, it is critical to understand that the chance of you individually benefiting from treatment is very small – usually quoted in the order of less than 5 per cent. One day, Sergei, who had endured a serious setback from a clinical trial, asked me why doctors would ever treat cancer with a drug that had no proven benefit and could even result in harm or death. But this is the key point – the drug is not offered for treatment, rather for experiment.

Drugs that are brought to Phase I have been studied by researchers on laboratory animals that are bred to produce specific tumours. Having seen encouraging results in the laboratory, a pharmaceutical company will elect to sponsor a clinical trial to see whether the results can be reproduced in human beings. A good clinical trial at a reputable centre is run under stringent conditions. The hospital ethics committee has to approve the trial as being fit to run on humans. The key investigators are trained in the use of the drug and its expected side effects. Every patient must sign a detailed consent form written in plain language. The trial coordinators keep a close eye on your progress. A blinded trial means that you will not know whether you are receiving an active substance or a placebo.

However, even if you are receiving an active drug you must understand that the very nature of early-phase trials means that you could experience unexpected side effects and possibly receive no benefit. This is because these trials are the medical profession's learning experience. Patients are very disappointed when they feel they 'discover the truth' about an early-phase clinical trial after their disease has become worse.

So should you ever participate in an early-phase trial? I think the answer is yes if you have talked things through with your doctor and understand what you are getting into. After all, even the most successful and established therapies began their journey with a trial, where doctors believed there was promise but the precise benefit remained unclear. It takes years of patience on behalf of the researchers, the altruism and goodwill of thousands of trial patients, and then decades of use, to realize both the potential and the side-effect profile of a new cancer drug. We owe enormous gratitude to patients who sacrifice their time and energy in order to help future generations. The truth is, by participating in an early-phase trial you are mainly helping future patients; you may receive incidental gains but the chances are very small. Being on such a trial generally won't make you live longer, although it may possibly alleviate some of your symptoms. Participation in early-phase trial is not simply about studying a drug, but also learning more about the behaviour of tumours. Trials require frequent doctors' visits and monitoring via blood tests and scans, or occasionally, biopsies. For some patients, this fulfils a curiosity, but many others find the frequent travelling and waiting tiresome and further tests invasive or painful.

So, at the very least, if you are thinking of enrolling in a clinical trial, it is worthwhile exploring the logistics first. Consider how physically robust you are to make frequent trips if they are needed; how prepared you are to undergo the tests demanded; and whether you have the necessary support structure, which may mean having a driver or an escort, finding accommodation close to the hospital, or any number of other things you may need help with. Ask yourself whether this is something that will bring you satisfaction and perhaps curb the regret of 'What if?' For some patients it is important to try absolutely everything they can get their hands on, but many others have had enough after standard therapies and simply want the treadmill to come to a stop, so that they can relish whatever time they have left. Temper your expectations and that of your relatives. Having a clear-eyed view of what an early-phase clinical trial will do for you and your family is really important.

If you don't like the sound of an early-phase trial, should you look for a Phase III clinical trial? Unlike its earlier counterparts, a Phase III trial is a more mature study of the effect of therapies that have successfully navigated the early-trial period. A Phase III trial is also known as a randomized controlled trial or a double-blind trial, which means that neither the doctor nor the patient knows whether a patient has been allocated to receive the new drug or the currently established or 'gold standard' therapy. Results of the drug can therefore be monitored without prior assumptions that one is better than the other. Some trials are conducted to prove that the new drug is non-inferior or simply as good as established drugs, while others are conducted in the hope of proving that the new treatment is better. Sometimes, the only way to access a promising new treatment is by enrolling in a clinical trial because the therapy is not yet publicly available. Some trials, but not all, allow 'crossover', which means that if you don't respond to your allocated treatment you may be switched over to another. In that case, if you were receiving the placebo, you may subsequently benefit from switching to the new drug.

All the logistical issues mentioned in relation to Phase I and Phase II trials also apply to Phase III. You still need to be physically robust, prepared to undergo frequent travel and tests, and understand that not all side effects of the new treatment are early or predictable. However, in view of the fact that the new drug has been under study for a longer time and has been filtered through the process of Phase I and Phase II trials, the potential benefit can be greater than that achieved by joining an early-phase trial. This is something that needs to be discussed in detail with your oncologist, who can advise you of the preliminary reports of the trial, the wider reaction of the oncology community to the practical usefulness of the therapy, and how other patients have fared on it. You should also read the consent form and plain-language explanation carefully and deliberately, and not hesitate to ask as many questions as you have. Far too many patients sign a document without questioning it. While it is reasonable to trust your oncologist to have your best interest at heart, and he or she does, it is you who are submitting yourself to research. Take the time to look into the nuances of your consent.

Clinical trial participation is abysmally low in many areas of cancer medicine. Less than 5 per cent of patients enrol in a trial so there is a continuing push for oncologists to encourage their patients to participate. Well-run trials are the only way we are going to make progress in the treatment of cancer. Depending on where you are being treated, there may be enthusiasm or reluctance about the subject. Academic hospitals usually have more trials open and more staff dedicated to recruiting patients, while a private practice or a small community hospital may not have the infrastructure to support trials. But regardless of whether your own hospital or oncologist participates, you have the right to seek advice about enrolling in a trial and your oncologist will help you by referring you to the right place.

Many patients demonstrate a remarkable sense of altruism by donating their precious time and energy to trials, thereby ensuring that future cancer sufferers will gain from the advances we make. Other patients derive personal health benefits from being part of a trial, which is gratifying not only for the patient but for doctors who learn from these experiences. The key to being a successful clinical trial participant, whether Phase I, II or III, is to understand what is on offer and how it best suits your goals of care.

Key Points

- A clinical trial is not necessarily treatment but an experiment that sets out to establish the value of a drug or intervention. Many trials do not result in successful drug development.
- The chance of direct individual benefit from an early-phase trial is minimal and your participation may mostly benefit future patients.
- A late-phase trial can offer you potential access to a useful treatment that is not commonly available; however, find out what the trial entails for you in terms of logistics, risk and benefit.
- Read the plain-language statement and never hesitate to ask questions.

14

What Happens Once I Finish Treatment?

If you have at last finished your cancer treatment you deserve congratulations. Even the strongest-willed patients describe having days when they doubted their ability to persevere. As an oncologist, I am often in awe of patients who put themselves through debilitating times to get through treatment.

As we have discussed, some people ultimately decide to stop treatment because it is no longer in their interest, or their hand is forced due to excessive side effects. Some people become too unwell to continue treatment, while others find their schedule constantly deferred, thus making chemotherapy seem like an endless ordeal. One patient's endless desire to persist with chemotherapy unfortunately never materialized because he was too weak to leave his hospital bed. So if you are someone who has managed to plough through a prescribed course of treatment within the predicted time frame you are entitled to experience pride and genuine relief.

You will surely notice now that the many blood tests have become less frequent, as have trips to hospital, crisis visits to the emergency room and the occasional admission to the busy wards. Gone are the long delays in the waiting room, knowing that if the oncologist is another few minutes late, the back pain will get worse or the vomiting won't wait.

Chemotherapy is usually a type of treatment that can stretch for months, or sometimes even longer. These days a few patients can even receive chemo or targeted therapy indefinitely. You may also have had radiotherapy, surgery, tablets and other interventions along the way. But for most patients, treatment, at least with chemo, will at some point come to a defined end.

Cancer cure rates are improving. Two-thirds of patients diagnosed with cancer now find themselves well five years on, and new treatments are keeping them well for even longer. So chances are looking up that you will find yourself in this fortunate position.

'It was a huge relief when I finished chemotherapy. My friends were sweet to throw me a party – it was wonderful to taste food again!' Relief and celebration are common at the end of treatment. The first or second anniversary of finishing treatment becomes a milestone, especially when there is no sign of recurrence. For many patients, being cancer-free at the three- or five-year mark is considered as good as a cure.

Patients often wonder when a cancer can be said to be beaten. 'It's been six years now. Can you now say if I'm in remission or do I still have to worry?' If your appendix has been removed, you can safely say that you will suffer no further attacks of appendicitis. If your gallbladder is out, the associated colic is happily a thing of the past. Your recovered ability to use your arm reassures you it is no longer broken. But in cancer, there are no absolutes. While the risk of recurrence may be statistically low, it is never zero.

Some patients recount anecdotes of a friend's cancer returning after decades, or of a neighbour developing a second cancer shortly after the first was successfully treated. While the chance of cancer recurrence does diminish with time, the knowledge that it could ever return causes universal anxiety. 'I don't care about dying if it comes back – what I dread are the tests, the travelling and all the emotional upheaval,' one patient said with a sigh. For another patient it was the waiting: 'It's the not-knowing that is so hard.'

Mild anxiety, especially in the early years after treatment, is quite normal. While you may relish the freedom from frequent consultations with the oncologist or long chemotherapy sessions, the end of these rituals also robs you of the security of close medical attention. Suddenly, no one is checking on your symptoms in detail, recording weight and blood pressure, looking at your swollen ankles or examining your wound regularly. No one is reminding you to fill your prescription or curb the alcohol. It's up to you to get to that annoying cough because there is no one to say, 'Let's just check it out while you are here.'

After perhaps feeling like your control was wrested away from you during diagnosis and treatment, all of a sudden the control is back in your hands whether you wanted it or not. Visits to the doctor have stretched out to every few months and the consultation time seems shorter now that it's not followed by a detailed chat with the chemo nurse, social worker or pharmacist. Many patients also realize – some to their dismay – that while patients receiving active chemotherapy have speedy access to doctors and nurses and emergency department help, the queue for other patients, including cancer survivors, is longer.

Surveillance after cancer therapy lasts anywhere between three and five years to much longer, depending on your circumstances. Your oncologist may still ask you to have a variety of periodic tests and scans. There is a growing recognition in the profession that many of these tests are not necessary, don't change your outcome, and in fact, result in accidental harm and needless anxiety. Oncologists' opinions on this vary. So if you are concerned that your friend's oncologist orders more tests than yours, don't fret but ask for an explanation. More is not always better. This is a good place to mention that not every patient requires the same type or duration of specialist follow-up. But if your specialist follow-up is about to end, you should expect to have a conversation about who is best placed to oversee your future care. It may be your family doctor, community nurses or another professional.

Worrying about test results is exceedingly common and although it decreases with time, for many patients it never disappears. 'I know it's silly, but I have sleepless nights all week before seeing you.' Some describe a rising sense of panic as the consultation day nears. This is normal. One way of containing anxiety and dealing with it effectively is to be a determined partner in your future care.

If you have never had the time or the energy to understand your disease and just wanted to focus on getting through treatment, the conclusion of treatment is a good time to review the basics with your oncologist. No question is too simple, no question is silly. Important things you may want to understand include how the cancer happened, where or how it was found and what treatment you had with what effect. If you have persisting side effects, are they expected to resolve and over what course of time? Damaged nerves heal very slowly but heartburn should improve quickly. Weakened muscles may take months to become stronger but nausea should vanish sooner. Ask if there is anything you can do to speed up recovery – ranging from gentle exercise and physical therapy to taking short-term medication for more troublesome symptoms. Find out if there is another professional you should see. For example, do you need a colonoscopy in one or two years? Should you keep seeing the psychologist? Is now a good time to see a physician about the heart trouble or high blood sugars you experienced during chemo? Does the surgeon need to see you to discuss breast reconstruction or the reversal of your colostomy bag? While patients feel that their oncologist should be across all these details and it should not be up to them to serve reminders, you are the best person to care about your health. Just prompting your oncologist helps him or her to think about your survivorship plan.

Some patients express frustration at not receiving proper explanations of the success of their treatment. 'I have no idea what my oncologist thinks. All I hear is that things look good. I have no idea whether that means my tumour has disappeared or shrunk, so I don't know what to tell my wife when she asks. But she says I need to pay more attention.' In order to avoid such frustration, you need to understand what your follow-up means. Ask your oncologist about which tests you will need and how frequently, what they reveal, and importantly, what they won't predict. As I have mentioned, abundant professional guidelines exist but an oncologist's individual practice varies depending on many factors, including your type of cancer, your age and coexisting illnesses. If you are receiving follow-ups with two or three different doctors – for example, a surgeon, oncologist and radiation therapist – check that all your tests are truly necessary and not being duplicated. Over-ordering and duplication of tests is a major problem, and it leads to inconvenience, cost and unnecessary stress. I would encourage you to check with your oncologist as to whether all planned tests are necessary. Unless there is a specific reason to see all your cancer doctors in a short span of time, arrange to see them in alternating fashion. Many patients see their oncologist and surgeon on an alternating basis for the first few years. Just as you would with your oncologist, it is perfectly reasonable to expect that your other specialists will provide an update to your family doctor; don't hesitate to remind them if you need to. Everyone knows that timely correspondence between health care professionals is sorely lacking.

For your care to smoothly transition between hospital and community, it is vital that your doctors communicate with each other. Having a good family doctor is always important but it becomes vital as your specialist appointments become infrequent. Your family doctor is the lynchpin in your complex medical care and the person who can coordinate the various players and keep track of them. The lack of correspondence between doctors is a vexed problem that family doctors in particular are affected by, because it diminishes their ability to provide seamless care. It is perfectly okay to remind your specialist to keep your doctor informed. If you have changed doctors, it's important that you let your specialists know. In any case, it's advisable to update your information from time to time. Sometimes correspondence can keep going to the wrong practitioner for months before someone corrects the error. You are entitled to your results, so if there are regular hiccups in communicating them to others, ask for a copy and keep a folder of your health records. Make an attempt to understand why certain tests are needed at certain times. It will help you comply with the tests and also feel more in control of your health.

'I know I should find a doctor but to be honest, I've never been sick in my life before this happened. And thankfully, I feel well again.' If you have never had or needed a primary-care doctor, the end of cancer treatment is a good time to find one. This is because you don't just need cancer follow-up but also attention to many other problems such as hypertension, weight management, diabetes, heart disease, cholesterol and osteoporosis. Your oncologist will manage your cancer but it's quite likely that if you have cancer, you have another health condition. It is not uncommon for patients to have meticulous management of their cancer while their non-cancer condition is ignored. But heart disease, pneumonia, diabetes, seizures or kidney disease can prove as serious as cancer – you still need to ensure that your vaccinations are up to date and that you are having the recommended health checks for your age and gender. I hope this convinces you that you need a regular doctor!

A common anxiety amongst cancer-treatment survivors is that the smallest symptom is a harbinger of cancer recurrence. 'Last night I was driving in the rain and my visibility was poor. All I could think was that the cancer had come back and affected my eyes. It's ridiculous, I know.' Every cold, muscle ache, or nosebleed raises suspicion. Every pain is cancer until proven otherwise, every rash is abnormal. If you have ever experienced cancer you will know how deep-seated this fear is. The good news is that most people are able to work their way through it and it improves with time, but if you think that your fear is crippling you and preventing you from leading a normal life, do seek professional advice. For some, opening up to your oncologist and seeking reassurance about symptoms may be enough. Others may require assistance from a psychologist or more informal conversations with a support group. Techniques that teach you how to handle the emotions and decisions associated with a cancer diagnosis could make all the difference to your quality of life.

The role of diet, exercise and weight management in survivorship is a perennial issue of interest. First of all, it is important to recognize that strict, randomized controlled trials – the so-called 'gold standard' of evidence – are lacking in this area, because it is notoriously difficult to control all the variables. However, there is increasing recognition that patients who make these kinds of lifestyle changes feel better physically and emotionally, experience less tiredness and possibly reduce their risk of recurrence of some cancers. The same goes for curbing habits such as smoking and drinking alcohol, which is never too late to do.

Although there is a multi-billion-dollar industry that promotes the use of dietary supplements and complementary therapy to manage nutrition and weight, there is no good evidence to date to suggest these things work unless you suffer from a specific nutritional deficiency, which is uncommon in well-nourished populations. The vast majority of patients just need to make a conscious effort to eat a healthy diet and perform moderate exercise, which, not surprisingly, is the same advice offered to everyone else in the general population.

A healthy diet is one that is high in fruits, vegetables and fibre and low in meats, sugars and heavily processed foods. Even healthy foods are a source of calories of course, so eat in moderation. I met a patient recently who took the advice to eat fruit so seriously that he consumed a whole watermelon every day. The resulting sugar load gave him severe diarrhoea and weight loss. You should avoid eliminating a particular food group altogether, or deviating from a healthy/balanced diet if you have existing dietary requirements, as this increases your chances of not obtaining essential nutrients. If you are concerned about your ability to distinguish the right foods or you don't know how much to eat, consult a dietician – adopting a sensible lifelong eating plan is turning out to be much more important than we ever thought.

As discussed later in Chapter 19, there is no single prescription for exercise – the important thing is to get some exercise in a form that is safe and enjoyable. You can start with a walk, swim, yoga or strength training without needing too much equipment or a trainer. It's important to exercise three or four times a week to improve fitness and flexibility. Doctors have always thought that exercise is beneficial, but evidence is now emerging that it may have some powerful effects on modifying the course of cancer recurrence.

It is never too late to quit smoking. If you have completed cancer treatment, smoking causes ongoing inflammation and an increased risk of developing a recurrence as well as a new cancer. Smoking is an addiction which is amenable to treatment but it also requires discipline.

Daily consumption of alcohol also has wide-ranging effects on disease recurrence and new cancers, not to mention the development of chronic liver disease and liver failure, potentially fatal in themselves. Most people have little idea of what a safe level of alcohol consumption means, so ask a doctor or nurse to take you through it.

It's important to point out that the relationship between modifying lifestyle factors and good health is not necessarily direct, and for every study that hints at an improvement in some aspect of your health there is another to contradict it. But recent years have shown a profusion of studies in cancer patients supporting the benefits of adopting a healthy lifestyle without going overboard. If you are unsure, ask your doctor, remembering that many patients never embark on these health measures because they are unsure whether they fit the bill and fear doing something that might hurt their health. It is important to discuss these kinds of concerns with your doctor. The relationship may be complex but weight management, exercise, curbing smoking and alcohol can have a positive influence on body image, self-confidence, anxiety, fatigue and quality of life. These are desirable aims in themselves.

Depression is common in cancer and its aftermath, as mentioned in the previous chapter. It may seem obvious that depression is likely to strike at the time of diagnosis and during cancer treatment, but patients and doctors sometimes forget that depression can become pronounced once the treatment rush is over and the reality of one's changed circumstances sets in. Therefore, it's important to be vigilant and treat depression promptly. Ongoing pain and fatigue, a delayed return to good health or great uncertainty about the future are all related to depression, as are poor social and emotional support structures. It may be useful to write down your most concerning symptoms. A clear explanation from your doctor may be sufficient to reduce anxiety and depression. Similarly, coming up with ways of addressing some of your most troublesome symptoms may ease emotional distress. Finally, you may need short- or long-term help from a psychologist or psychiatrist to tackle depression. The key is to identify depression and seek help without feeling stigmatized.

Along the way, as a survivor you may also face issues to do with your relationships, fertility, work and so on. These are matters that we all tackle in life but your circumstances may be altered by your cancer experience. Many patients expect that people around them, especially those who are close, will understand their plight and support them unconditionally. But just as having cancer is confronting, for many people so is being near it. Some of your closest friends and family might feel that your experience represents their own near-brush with mortality. Others can't cope with the mental or physical strain of being a carer or a friend. Some relationships break down due to financial stress. Being a cancer patient is difficult but being in a relationship with one can be testing too. Sometimes there just isn't enough understanding to go around. But be hopeful, things will generally start to look up and many couples and families not only survive the experience but emerge stronger from it.

'If I begin to tell you the ways in which cancer has affected my life, we'll be here all day, doctor. I feel like someone broke me into pieces but couldn't manage to put me back together properly.'

Cancer treatment may have altered or completely overturned your plans for pregnancy or parenthood, which is a sensitive and special matter at the best of times. You may have taken up your doctor's advice on fertility preservation, or perhaps there was no time to think about it or it wasn't even recommended. Oncologists have been known to tell some high-risk patients bluntly that they should put the matter of having children behind them. The task of coping with cancer may have been all-consuming, diverting your attention from your children, elderly parents or others. The resulting detachment can be hard to patch up, especially if you feel guilty or are still working through your own symptoms.

Some workplaces are very sympathetic and accommodating, whereas others have to let go of chronically ill employees due to workforce pressures. Many patients resign their jobs under pressure. Others can't tolerate what they say is thinly veiled impatience on the part of their colleagues. 'I overheard someone saying to the boss, "It's not my fault she got cancer. Why should I have to work harder?"'

Your oncologist may proclaim you well but you don't feel well enough to return to work. You may be upset by your altered looks, that your clothes don't fit, or that the cancer has made you re-examine your priorities. 'My secretary was groaning about a minor cold and it took me all my self-control to remind her that I nearly died from cancer.'

These are just some of the issues my patients tell me about what happens during survivorship. Survivors face a long list of issues that they must work through, often with poor recognition and minimal support. 'Everyone thinks I'm lucky to be alive but my life feels like a wreck,' a young chef observed, after her cancer treatment. Her husband of five years left and she lost her job due to the nerve damage that prevented the free use of her hands. It took her three years to recover from the emotional trauma and to retrain in another role. Then, she said, 'I was so fragile. I wish I had believed in myself, been less impatient and forgiven myself more.'

I think this is a good message to leave you with. Survivorship is exhilarating, something that people are enormously grateful for, but there can be bumps ahead. Expect them, be patient, work through the problems, seek help, and most of all, have faith that things will improve. Good luck.

Key Points

- More and more patients are surviving their cancer diagnosis and are facing survivorship issues.
- Not all side effects subside quickly after the end of chemotherapy. Speak to your doctor and find out what to expect in the aftermath.
- Looking after your diet and exercise, and emotional health are just some of the things you can do to stay well after cancer treatment.
- Many patients realize the full extent of their ordeal once treatment finishes. Talk to your oncologist about ways to maintain good physical and emotional health.

15

I'm Getting Worse – What Is the Best Course?

I met Jack when he was diagnosed with pancreatic cancer in his seventies. It was discovered quite incidentally when he came in for a hip repair for bad osteoarthritis. He underwent a successful hip replacement but his cancer was inoperable. He was sent to me for advice about chemotherapy. Jack was a fit man who regularly played cricket with a seniors' team that had been together since the men became first-time parents and bonded over the group. Jack was keen to start treatment as soon as possible so that he could get back to bowling and doing the other things he enjoyed with his family. He and his wife, Sally, lived on a small farm at the edge of town where his grandchildren visited them most weekends. The visits were something the whole family looked forward to.

We discussed the fact that since diagnosis Jack had become aware of a mild discomfort in his abdomen and didn't feel much like eating. Sally thought he had lost a few pounds but other than that, Jack was well. He started chemotherapy and, somewhat unexpectedly for pancreatic cancer, had an extraordinary response. The cancer shrunk and his symptoms settled. His bowling club had just resumed, so Jack and I together decided to stop treatment. It wasn't until nine months later that he began experiencing pain, and scans showed cancer growth. He readily resumed chemotherapy and this time had to cope patiently with the side effects for some months before we saw a response. When the response reached a plateau, that is, ongoing chemotherapy did not reduce the cancer or improve his symptoms, he decided on another break from treatment. He was very tired and just didn't feel as spirited as he did the first time around. I supported his idea of taking a break to enjoy his farm.

I worried about the next round of chemotherapy, and my concern was answered by his reappearance only two months later with more pain and fatigue. Scans showed that the cancer was on the march yet again, this time to local lymph glands and his liver. We discussed that although he had had a remarkable response for a year and a half, this time things looked more serious. He was disappointed but, determined to do something, he embarked on a third round of treatment. He said that he was mindful his constitution the first time around had been the strongest, the second round had tested him, and that the third was likely to be worse, but he still felt encouraged to try. As an oncologist, whenever patients receive multiple rounds of treatment separated by time, my greatest concern is to ensure that their expectation moves with their circumstances. Jack assured me that he understood each successive round of chemotherapy had a smaller chance of working. We eventually started chemotherapy but he began struggling almost immediately. Having turned eighty recently, he said he could feel the slowing done in his bones. He experienced severe nausea and fatigue. His pain levels fluctuated – well controlled one week, but troublesome the next, often without a trigger. Eating became a chore, done more out of obligation to his wife Sally than any real interest.

He was travelling nearly two hours to see me because he valued our existing relationship, but I could see that my once amiable and jocular patient had lost his spark. I watched him become increasingly dependent on Sally to remember the details of his symptoms and medications, but he was also irritable at the loss of control. If I directed a question to Sally, he would say sharply, 'I can answer that myself!'. But actually he was often unable to, getting mixed up with the days, doses and other details. Sally would patiently rescue him by pretending to consult their diary when she knew by heart the answers to my questions.

Suspecting his advancing cancer to be the culprit, I arranged for Jack to have a CT scan. To my surprise, its appearance had not altered dramatically. 'I can see a lot of disease, Jack, but I can't say it looks worse than two months ago.' Hearing this, Jack asked to push on with treatment. I was caught in a dilemma because I had already made up my mind that the chemo was making him feel worse. However, his enthusiasm swayed me and I set about to manage his symptoms more aggressively. Unfortunately, altering Jack's pain medication and adjusting some of his other tablets did little to change the general nature of how he felt. He would be fine for a week or two and then have three bad weeks where he felt weak, irritable and unwell. Chemotherapy, which I kept wanting to stop, was frequently deferred and the nurses began to wonder why I kept bringing him back for more when the writing was on the wall. Then Jack got pneumonia and spent two weeks in hospital, emerging from this serious setback feeling very weak. Although we only had faint expectations of it, he got back on his feet and for a while looked like his old self, only thinner. Again, he insisted on resuming chemotherapy, which I did at a much lower dose after asking him to think about his decision for a week. 'I want to go down fighting' was his typical response.

But Jack was back within the next fortnight. 'I don't get it,' he said, with exasperation. 'If the cancer is stable, how can I feel worse each time?'

Another exhaustive look at his general health and his drug list didn't reveal anything we were not addressing.

'Jack,' I said, finally, 'I think it's your cancer. While there is no single drug or symptom responsible for your feeling bad, the cancer burden is plenty to make you feel tired and unwell. I want you to really think about whether having chemotherapy is exacerbating everything. I suspect it is, but only you can confirm it.' After a pause I added gently, 'Jack, it may be time to stop chemo.'

'But what happens if he stops?' Sally asked. 'He'll just get worse, won't he?'

I could see Sally's reluctance to stopping a treatment that was seemingly doing him good. But from my objective vantage point I saw Jack thinner, weaker and less interested in life. The chemotherapy would not prolong his life and I really wanted him to enjoy some quality before he became ill again.

'How your tumour appears on a scan is only one small aspect of your overall care, Jack,' I explained. 'You're looking and feeling unwell, and today you can barely stay awake for our short consultation. I'd really like you to think about the future.

Sally nodded. 'I'm beginning to feel that we should stop. I can see that it's making him worse.' Her husband stared at the floor in glum agreement.

When Jack and Sally returned three weeks later I was glad to see him looking better than on many previous occasions. He was in a decisive mood. 'Doctor, I am here to tell you that I have had enough. I'm becoming weaker and sicker and I don't want to die chasing a scan that looks good.'

I agreed that based on his overall poor experience, the time had indeed come to stop chemotherapy for good and concentrate on quality of life. Jack spent the next two months free of travelling to the clinic, blood tests and scans. There was a short period when he felt well enough to be wheeled to the bowling club from where he cheered on his team – their fondness for him always buoyed his spirits.

Jack slowly declined, was admitted to hospice and died peacefully a few days later. In a phone call, his wife Sally sounded so content that I commented on her positive attitude. 'It's because I know that he had a good life and made the right decision,' she said. 'I don't worry that he stopped chemotherapy earlier than he liked because these two months were the perfect end. He spent them doing the things he loved.'

All patients can feel when they are becoming worse. Patients sense their deterioration earlier and more accurately than their doctors but many are afraid of saying so because they fear the consequences. Some are desperate to continue chemotherapy, while others don't want to upset their loved ones. It is the uncommon patient who takes matters into their own hands to put an end to active treatment. But stopping chemotherapy doesn't mean stopping care – in fact it means the opposite. It means actively deciding to pursue quality of life when chemotherapy is not achieving its goals.

Patients assume that if chemotherapy isn't working, their doctor will tell them. This might lead to a change of drugs or other helpful measures not previously tried, or perhaps even the possibility of entering a clinical trial. No oncologist wants a patient to undergo futile chemotherapy. The problem is that words like 'value' and 'futile' are difficult to define for an individual patient, due to widely varying philosophies of life. For example, while Jack decided against having chemotherapy, another patient may have taken the same set of tests to indicate that he was responding to treatment and hence needed to continue it for as long as possible. Such a patient might have accepted poor quality of life as a fact of receiving chemotherapy and roused himself from his bed for every chemotherapy visit, before returning to convalesce in bed. A disheartening number of patients receiving palliative chemotherapy, that is chemotherapy for incurable disease, will do this because they feel stuck. It is critical for the oncologist, nurses, carers and the patient to be aware that this happens.

Jack was not so critically ill that giving chemo was definitively the wrong thing to do, so in the absence of a clear directive from him, it would not be unusual to continue treatment in fits and starts. But this would almost certainly have led to a serious event forcing my hand to stop chemotherapy altogether. As a patient it can often be up to you whether you want to wait for a critical event or make a pre-emptive decision that you have had enough. I don't say this lightly because I imagine it is one of the most burdensome decisions for a patient to make. In my experience, when the oncologist alone makes the decision to stop chemotherapy, a patient can feel let down. But sometimes waiting for the patient to realize that chemotherapy is doing harm can lead to more harm.

Some patients, like Jack, find that their situation fluctuates so much that they can't be sure if they are really getting worse. Their good weeks make them forgiving of the bad ones and they wait for something grave to happen. But many other patients fear that openly accepting that they are becoming sicker will become a self-fulfilling prophecy and that if they no longer have chemotherapy they will let themselves and other people down. In my experience, this is a common reason people put up with many onerous interventions when they are ill.

You should never persevere with toxic treatment by deluding yourself about its benefits to you or others. You are the person who must endure the inconvenience and harm, you shoulder all the side effects although your carers might be sympathetic towards you, and your own observation about your health is the most meaningful. You may have difficulty understanding why you feel sick, especially if you hear conflicting medical opinions, but deep down, you know when something isn't right. Heed this change in your well-being. I suggest you write down your observations and share them with your oncologist or a nurse who is familiar with your progress. Sometimes, consultations are short and you'll feel you don't have enough time to discuss this important subject. If possible, plan ahead and signal your intention clearly. Bring someone along who knows you, and can back up your concerns and offer support. Remember that if you consistently feel yourself deteriorating, chances are it's true. Give yourself an opportunity to feel better.

Key Points

- If you feel you are getting worse, you almost certainly are. Discuss this with your oncologist; don't wait for someone to raise it with you.
- Write down your most troublesome symptoms so that you can remember them during a consultation. Bring someone along who is familiar with your deterioration and can add helpful details.
- Don't continue toxic treatment for the sake of other people; it is better to safeguard quality of life.

16

Managing Pain

'I'm used to having cancer and I'm not afraid of dying, but what keeps me awake at night is the thought of dying in pain.'

If you are like most patients I'm sure the subject of pain has crossed your mind. No assumption, and no fear, is more closely associated with cancer than having pain. And while it is true that many patients with cancer experience pain at some stage, the good news is that many others don't. Western countries are also fortunate in having ready access to strong painkillers such as morphine. However, it's human nature to fear bad outcomes and disregard positive ones.

Let me reassure you that modern methods and new drugs mean we can treat cancer pain more effectively than ever before. Unfortunately, though, pain remains one of the most under-treated symptoms of cancer – hence the purpose of this chapter is to help you understand and navigate your pain management.

I met a patient recently who was diagnosed with cancer nearly nine months ago. She was simultaneously diagnosed with a neurological condition that had left her weak in the legs and necessitated a move to a nursing home. She was too weak to receive chemotherapy but was referred to me for periodic follow-up. Before inviting her into my room I viewed her original scans, which showed widespread disease. The scans looked ominous and as I prepared to usher her in, I imagined a crippled patient and readied my script pad while paging the palliative-care nurse in anticipation. But when the patient arrived she looked well, calm and certainly not in pain. I surreptitiously double-checked her particulars to make sure I had the right patient. As she took her seat, I assumed that she indeed had pain but it was so well managed that she was having a good day. But this too turned out to be untrue. No, she told me smilingly, she didn't have any pain whatsoever and her biggest obstacle was in fact the weakness in her legs preventing her from walking. Her case was a gratifying and salient reminder that not all cancers that look aggressive behave so, and not every cancer patient experiences pain.

You may be troubled by pain or discomfort at various points. Commonly, it happens in the phase leading up to diagnosis. For a sizeable number of patients, it can take weeks or months to come to a diagnosis of cancer, and an experience of pain might well be attributed to a variety of other causes first. After all, you are more likely to be troubled by arthritis, a sports injury, a benign backache or sciatica than cancer, leading many patients to initially receive a recommendation of a combination of rest, mild painkillers and physiotherapy. Even if the pain does not go away, it is often temporarily alleviated and this can be reassuring enough to delay further tests. Contrary to popular belief, cancer pain can also have peaks and troughs and doesn't always worsen with time.

However, if the pain returns and is troublesome, suspicion may be aroused of a rather more problematic cause. Again, the nature of medical consultation means significant time may elapse before more intensive tests are done. What can be frustrating is that even when a diagnosis of cancer becomes apparent, the rush to confirm the diagnosis and arrange for the numerous associated tasks means that patients can miss out on proper pain management. It took one of my patient two months to be diagnosed with multiple myeloma, and in that time, while numerous doctors advised her of their suspicion of cancer, her actual pain management somehow always took the last seat.

Something similar happened to another patient who was injured in a minor boating accident. She attributed her back and leg pain to a pulled muscle and took all reasonable measures at home for four months before her family doctor astutely picked up that something wasn't right. Her greatest relief on being diagnosed with cancer – if there was one – was that she came off the anti-inflammatory drugs she had been swallowing around the clock in sufficient quantity to give herself a peptic ulcer.

Pain can also develop during the term of having cancer, affecting either an internal organ or bones. Pain from an internal organ, such as the liver or lymph glands, is usually experienced as *referred* pain; that is, it's located on an *outside* part of the body, due to the way the nervous system works. Cancer pain may be sporadic or continuous. Nerve pain is described as sharp, electrical jolts. Bone pain can be deep-seated. One person's pain can simply be another's discomfort, and vice versa.

Many patients find it enormously frustrating to be interrogated by a doctor about pain. Doctors can ask seemingly tedious questions, such as what it feels like, when it started, where it goes, what makes it worse, and whether anything helps. When your doctor asks these questions they can sound seemingly irrelevant if you are fed up with the trouble, but your answers help to tailor your pain management.

On a good morning, it can be hard to remember all the details of a painful day. So I advise my patients to jot down some of the features of their pain when they notice it. Is there a pattern to it? For example, does it occur with movement or rest? Is it in one spot or all over? Do you always wake up a few hours after going to bed or is it more a problem in the early morning? Are evenings better or mornings? If you are groaning at these questions, understand that sometimes the truth is that it can be quite difficult to categorize cancer pain and it seems to come in as many forms as there are patients. Some people find the pain exacerbated by certain movements, others feel it's worse at a particular time, while a small proportion of patients suffer continuous pain that is very hard to manage. It's not possible to accurately predict which type of pain you will have and for how long. You also can't always be sure what is hurting, especially if cancer affects more than one body part.

More than any sophisticated test, considered, comprehensive answers to the above questions go a long way towards helping your doctor manage your pain. For example, it may be that simply switching your medication to the right time intervals will do the trick. Or your doctor may discover that you are not taking the correct amount of medication. Alternatively, it may become quickly apparent that your current mix of painkillers is not right for you.

While some pain is genuinely difficult to control, a large number of cases are simply inadequately managed. The reason for this is twofold. First, as people are living longer, the need to manage all kinds of pain is increasing. Many doctors graduate with only basic knowledge in the area, or find themselves behind in the recent advances in pain management and knowledge of new drugs available. Doctors specializing in pain management or pain clinics are not widely accessible, so cancer patients most commonly turn to their family doctor or oncologist to treat pain. If these doctors do not or cannot manage pain properly, a patient can experience pain for unacceptable lengths of time. Fortunately, more and more doctors are recognizing the importance of learning good pain management skills.

To me, another common reason for cancer patients experiencing pain is the most regrettable – the patient's failure to report pain accurately to the doctor. 'Why didn't you tell me you had pain?' I once asked a young woman wincing in her chemotherapy chair. Her nurse had summoned me after picking up that the patient was not sleeping well at night. 'I figured you knew,' she said. 'And anyway, everyone with my condition has pain so I just have to accept it.' There is a widespread assumption by patients that pain is just part and parcel of having cancer and it is pointless complaining. Does this sound familiar to you? If so, please believe me that it's not true.

While pain frequently accompanies cancer, much of it can be adequately controlled. If you can't tolerate tablets, there are patches. If patches are not your thing, there are lozenges. There are also any variety of injections, depot injections that deliver drugs over time, capsules, dissolvable drugs and nerve blocks. There really is something for everyone, so don't give up. Every year sees new developments and fresh insights gained into pain management, so it's critical that you tell your doctor you have pain and expect it to be addressed. I have a young patient who had a very difficult time controlling pain as a result of radiation-induced damage to her abdomen. She didn't want to come to hospital because of her young children, Hence, for a time, I asked her to call me every week with an update. She said she felt like a nuisance but I insisted that her report, good or bad, reassured me of her condition. It took time but eventually her pain improved. So if your doctor or nurse asks you to check in with them frequently, don't feel bad, accept the offer.

If you have already tried some painkillers and found them unhelpful, instead of dismissing them as useless, spend some time determining how they're failing. Ask someone who lives with you whether they can help you pick up any patterns. For example, a medication might provide good relief but not last long enough, in which case its dose, formulation or the frequency can be changed rather than the drug itself. Or another medication might produce all the expected side effects without doing much for your pain, in which case it is best to abandon it before your troubles mount. Many people don't realize that no matter how many pills they take, it is not the correct management of their pain if the pills are actually ineffective.

You may have noticed that a patch is more convenient for you than tablets. Some people find it troublesome to swallow large pills but don't mind liquid versions. You may find that without treatment your pain is okay when you are resting but that doing anything strenuous is impossible, in which case medication can be timed for slightly before you begin an activity, to help get you through it. The bottom line is that just like chemotherapy, modern pain relief comes in many forms. Admittedly, even having all this information at hand still doesn't provide an instant fix, but the more information you can give your doctor the more you are helping your cause.

Remember that requirements for pain relief or reduction can and often do change – what worked last month may not be good enough this month or the next. Similarly, being on a high dose of painkillers one month doesn't mean you are consigned to it for the rest of your life. Fluctuations in pain are normal and need to be discussed with the doctor who manages your pain. You may have reservations about broaching the same problem repeatedly, but mentioning recurrent or persisting pain is perfectly normal and expected.

If you feel that your current doctor is not managing your pain adequately, you might politely suggest that you would like to see someone else. Depending on where you live, you may have access to a specialized pain clinic, an anaesthetist or a palliative-care doctor. This doesn't mean you will constantly have to see another doctor, which many patients find onerous. Your usual doctor may comfortably monitor the regimen a specialist has prescribed. But seeing someone else once or twice can go a long way towards better symptom management. Do keep in mind that the option of palliative care may be appropriate for you. We will talk about this a little later in the book.

In some situations, chemotherapy or radiotherapy may be appropriate for addressing pain. Chemotherapy circulates throughout the bloodstream and therefore has a wide effect. If effective, it works by shrinking cancerous masses that are causing pain, either by direct pressure or by producing signals in the bloodstream. But as we have discussed elsewhere, chemotherapy is associated with a number of side effects that have to be taken into account. Certain patients experience pain due to high calcium levels in the bloodstream; for them, lowering the calcium level provides effective relief.

Radiotherapy is focused on a few specific areas of pain. Radiation is particularly effective for targeting bony pain but it is also used for other reasons in consultation with the specialist. A recent patient I saw was experiencing discomfort from a bleeding rectal cancer. Local radiation stemmed the bleeding and pain. Individual organs are affected differently by radiotherapy and your radiation oncologist will advise you if radiotherapy is feasible and what side effect to anticipate. If you have previously met a radiation oncologist, you can return to discuss management of your pain. Alternatively, if you have never met one, your oncologist can refer you.

Some patients reluctantly confess that they fear if they start taking strong drugs such as morphine too early in the course of the illness, their body will stop responding to it when they really need it. This understandably makes many people worry about the right time to start morphine because they don't want to be in pain later on in life. Another common fear is that by taking morphine, patients will turn into drug addicts. Allow me to reassure you that these are myths. While the body can develop tolerance to a drug, which means higher doses may be required with time, it's unusual to stop responding to morphine and its equivalents altogether. And when used for a legitimate purpose such as cancer pain, use of morphine will not turn you into a drug addict. This is because true pain is probably associated with different mechanisms of drug action than when drugs are used to seek pleasure.

As our understanding of pain has evolved, we know that instead of following the formerly recommended drug 'ladder', where doctors learned to always prescribe milder drugs before stronger ones, it is sometimes more useful to simultaneously prescribe a few drugs with different modes of action. So for example, your doctor may prescribe a small dose of morphine, an anti-inflammatory and a steroid to stabilize your pain quickly. Some of these drugs may then be reduced or escalated, depending on response.

This practice allows potent drugs to be delivered in smaller doses and it makes sense to target more than one pain pathway. It doesn't mean that everyone needs to start with strong drugs; in fact, the general principle is still sound that you should only take the medications you really need and the ones that have the least side effects.

Many people with cancer do end up on morphine and related drugs, such as fentanyl and hydromorphone, classed together as opioids. Opioids are easily available in rich countries and come in a number of formulations, which means they can be adapted to many needs. For a lucky few, they do not cause side effects, but unfortunately, many people experience unwanted problems. Sometimes, these improve with time as the body becomes used to the drug. But some patients find the nausea, sleepiness, constipation or lack of attentiveness persistent and troubling. If your pain is well controlled, your doctor might try to manage these side effects with other medications. That means taking more pills but you may find nausea or constipation easier to tackle or tolerate than pain. Many people reluctantly accept a reduction in their attention span or mental sharpness but feel that they would rather be pain-free in the hours that they are awake. Just like pain relief itself there are many potent medications to combat its side effects.

Just as it's important to increase pain medications when needed, it is critical to review the ongoing need for powerful drugs. Many patients observe that once they have been started on morphine, doctors are reluctant to stop them. But if you are lucky enough to be entirely pain-free for a substantial length of time, it is reasonable to try to wean drugs. Some patients have managed to come off these drugs entirely and gained a better quality of life, so don't be afraid to try. An elderly lady with breast cancer on large doses of fentanyl balked when I first suggested reducing the dose. To her amazement, she came off the drug completely in six weeks and gained herself a less foggy mind in the process.

The key thing about pain is that you don't simply have to put up with it and that you know to seek help. It's okay to report changes regularly, expect authoritative help with pain and expect ongoing adjustments to your regimen as your condition changes. Be as clear as possible about the nature of your pain. By working together, you and your oncologist will most likely find acceptable ways to ease your pain.

Key Points

- Many patients experience pain during cancer: it is common, under-recognized and under-managed. Never hesitate to discuss pain.
- Uncontrolled pain as part of having cancer is not acceptable.
- Modern pain management is greatly advanced and can be tailored to your situation.
- Not all doctors are confident in managing pain. It can require different experts, time and patience. Ask for help in finding a pain specialist if you think you need one.

17

How Cancer Affects Appetite, Diet and Weight

Cancer patients and their loved ones are forced to become used to any number of changes in their life. Perhaps you initially disbelieved you had cancer and you have had to come to terms with the diagnosis, as well as helping those close to you towards acceptance. If you once prided yourself on avoiding doctors you may realize that you see more of them now than your own family. From routines and interests, to travel plans and employment, nothing escapes change during cancer treatment, and I am always impressed and humbled to see how well and how graciously most people cope with change.

However, one of the hardest things to come to terms with is the change in food habits. Practically every patient is affected at some point by a positive or negative change in appetite, and fluctuation in their weight. Some people, especially when they are receiving chemotherapy, find they have a voracious appetite while others suffer the opposite problem. Just as in everyday life, food and weight are thorny topics in cancer too.

If you have heard a dozen opinions on what kind of cancer therapy you should be having, I don't need to tell you that there are many, many more opinions about what you should be eating to beat your cancer. A routine part of my day involves discussing the advice that patients bring in, which ranges from the conflicting and confusing to the ill-advised and downright dangerous.

An early, but by no means universal, sign of cancer can be a loss of appetite and weight, which many patients realize in hindsight when reflecting on the period leading up to their diagnosis. These days, so many of us are overweight and unfit that we are usually pleased to shed a few kilos.

Weight loss in cancer is pathological; that is, it happens despite you trying to maintain a healthy weight. The loss occurs because cancers consume a lot of energy to fuel their own growth, so in a way, the disease is taking away your resources.

Before discussing weight loss let me touch briefly on weight gain, which is a particular problem while having some types of chemotherapy. It is especially common in women undergoing treatment with chemotherapy or hormonal therapy for breast cancer, when a gain of 10 to 20 kilograms may occur. But patients on other treatments can also experience this problem. Steroids, commonly prescribed with chemotherapy to avoid nausea and vomiting, are a key culprit. Steroids promote appetite and cause people to eat more than they would usually. Sometimes you can cut back on the steroids to avoid putting on weight, but it is not possible or recommended for everyone.

Fatigue, muscle deconditioning and a lack of initiative to exercise also cause weight gain. It is common to make up for emotional trauma by eating more and selecting unhealthy choices as comfort foods.

'I want to look good after finishing chemo, but I'm embarrassed by my weight and dread the long road to getting fit again,' one patient explained. Weight gain is associated with lack of self-esteem and a host of other problems. However, there are sensible ways to achieve a healthy weight and we will discuss them in a separate chapter that deals with issues of survivorship and staying well.

Weight loss is the more common issue with cancer. 'I met a lady who can't lose weight after chemo. I wish I had her problem. The nurse tells me that if I don't stop losing weight the doctors might have to reconsider my chemo.' Unfortunately, weight loss is a very visible problem, especially in the latter stages of illness when people routinely complain that their weight is falling off despite their conscious effort to eat more. 'All my life I have wanted to be small – now I crave some fat to cushion me,' one lady sighed. A bachelor who doubted his own cooking abilities and arranged for a healthy meals delivery programme observed, 'These are the best meals I have ever had but you wouldn't know to look at me. My clothes are hanging off me.'

Almost every chemotherapy patient at some point describes intolerance to certain smells and textures, prominent nausea associated with meals, or simply a lack of interest in food, even previously favourite meals. Sometimes there is an obvious barrier, such as pain during swallowing, a persistent sense of fullness, vomiting or the risk of exacerbating abdominal discomfort or a bowel obstruction. Other patients lack the will to prepare food or cannot sustain the energy to sit down for a full meal.

If you are nauseous this week, it doesn't mean that you will be the same next week. If you have been restricted to no solid food for the last few days due to a bowel obstruction it doesn't mean you will never eat properly again. But the changes do mean that you eat and absorb food unpredictably, exposing you to fluctuations in weight.

'I don't care what else he does, doctor, but tell him to eat like a regular man,' a feisty Italian wife once said, chiding her husband in my clinic. The patient was well known in his clan to relish the multi-course meals she lovingly made, but lately she couldn't spark his interest in eating. 'I can't tell her,' he groaned privately, 'but just the smell of her cooking makes me feel ill. I can't bear to see it. All I want is a dry biscuit, but that sounds so ungrateful.'

Few things cause more anxiety to the patient, and even more so to loved ones, than a patient's loss of appetite and the associated weight loss. On one hand, unlike nausea or pain, weight loss is a visibly upsetting reminder of cancer, and on the other, food is much more than a means of meeting the body's nutritional needs – it is interwoven in our culture. We eat to celebrate. Families who don't do much else together will still join hands over a meal. Food celebrates our togetherness and our curiosity for exploration. It nourishes and comforts. Who can't remember a time when sitting down to a favourite meal has alleviated stress and afforded us temporary distraction? Important family events are marked by an abundance of food. In normal circumstances, our spirits lift at the sight of food and few things are as comforting as a hearty meal.

It is hard for sick patients, but even harder for their healthy carers to reconcile to the fact that food no longer feels special. You may find that as a patient, you come to a quick acceptance that you aren't interested in food, or that it brings on unwelcome effects such as nausea, pain or bloating. But your relatives might struggle to reach a similar understanding. It can be genuinely difficult for others to fathom how someone cannot find anything appealing from a parade of choices.

One husband tried everything to interest his wife in food but to no avail. He can't understand why, despite every doctor and dietician encouraging her to gain weight, she won't indulge herself. 'Okay, she can't stand mashed vegetables or broth but how can she deny a bar of smooth chocolate or rich ice cream for lunch? She has a free pass!'

'I have given up trying to explain,' his wife sighed. 'He is so intent on feeding me that he will never understand why I don't enjoy his favourite creations, but I just can't taste anything. I *hate* food.'

Cooking for someone is a gesture of concern, affection and goodwill. Family members and friends go to great lengths to buy special books and unearth novel recipes for cancer patients. They go in search of fresh and exotic ingredients and purchase unique and costly food and equipment to maximize the benefit. Somebody who previously never spent hours in the kitchen adopts meticulous planning and diligent cooking. You can see why your carers are disappointed or even annoyed when your enthusiasm doesn't match theirs. Patients tell me that they feel they are being ungrateful or not trying hard enough to please their carers. But this is not true, and it can be helpful to understand why somebody with cancer does not experience appetite, hunger or pleasure in eating in the same way as a normal healthy person.

Cancer triggers many complex hormones and ill-understood mechanisms to suppress your appetite. The mere presence of cancer, even without chemotherapy added, can cause nausea and suppress appetite. Scientists think that alterations in appetite and weight regulation take place at various levels including in muscle, fat, the immune system and the brain itself. There are so many different cells and biological pathways involved that we don't yet understand them fully, although this is an increasingly active area of research for its widespread implications.

All forms of cancer therapy, from chemotherapy and radiation to hormones, can cause suppression of appetite, loss of taste, nausea and weight change. Nausea is one of the commonest side effects of chemotherapy and many patients find it exacerbated by the very sight of food. You might feel a constant tug or churning in your abdomen, which you don't want to provoke by eating. While nausea can be especially pronounced in the immediate aftermath of chemotherapy, regrettably some patients suffer from a more persistent form of it.

Chemotherapies can be graded according to the nausea and vomiting they induce, but even then, your individual sensitivity to the drug is not always immediately predictable. It is reasonable to assume that if you felt intensely nauseous after your first one or two cycles, you will need aggressive treatment for nausea for the rest. Chemotherapy, targeted therapy and radiotherapy to the head, neck or face area can lead to destruction of the taste buds in the tongue. 'Everything tastes metallic' is one of the most common complaints I hear. In fact, many patients are so resigned to it that they don't even bother mentioning it unless asked.

Many patients also require powerful painkillers, including morphine and related drugs. These painkillers are effective but they have their own list of significant side effects, with nausea and constipation being prominent. Any number of other drugs, including commonly prescribed antibiotics, can cause nausea. Nausea can also result from pain.

Other eating problems can come from oral thrush as a result of immune suppression from cancer and chemotherapy, which can limit your enjoyment of food. Constipation is also widely prevalent in cancer, caused by morphine-like drugs, chemotherapy, lack of dietary fibre and fluid and relative immobility. You might notice that constipation becomes a prolonged battle, resulting in intense nausea and lack of appetite. Other transient problems that patients experience include painful mouth ulcers, hiccupping and disturbed swallowing, all of which contribute to a lack of desire to eat.

This is not an all-inclusive list but I hope it helps you and your loved ones understand that there are numerous reasons you may not feel like eating. It can be hard to finely separate them all and expect that resolving each problem will add up to a solution. Certainly, treating obvious pain, mouth ulcers, nausea or constipation is important for their own sake. But you may find that sometimes this still won't achieve the goal of weight maintenance or arresting weight loss. It may be a sign of an overall deterioration in your condition. It could imply that your illness is using more energy than you can put in. You are in an uneven match, the kind that cancer often poses. Talk to your oncologist or another doctor about it if nothing seems to be working.

If you are a family member helplessly watching this take place, you are not alone. A consistently painful experience for carers is witnessing someone you care about deteriorate before your eyes.

'I just want you to tell me how to help him. Is there anything I can do?' a wife pleaded with me. The most important thing you can give a patient in this situation is your understanding. I can reassure you that while the decline can be uncomfortable to watch, it is normal, a part and parcel of having cancer. Avoid making the patient feel as if he is being obstructive or disrespectful by turning down your offering. Allow him the freedom to eat what he chooses and when. It is best not to be prescriptive about food. A full and balanced meal is often not possible. I often advise patients to graze on small amounts and not feel compelled to finish a meal or have three full meals a day.

While it's ideal to eat nutritious foods, especially if you are not managing regular meals, many people forget that enjoyment is also important. It's no use pressing cheese, eggs, milk and fruit on someone who is repulsed by their sight. It's better to enjoy a few spoons of ice cream than nothing at all. Supplemental energy bars and protein-rich drinks are okay if you can tolerate them, but many patients find that they lack taste and resent being forced to turn to them. If you're looking after somebody who is having a hard time with these supplements, you can help them with an understanding word and perhaps even by encouraging them to have a break.

When a cancer patient's ability to eat really drops off, often in the final few weeks or days of life, there is often a flurry of activity by concerned relatives. Some of my prolonged and most painful consultations involve families pleading for doctors to start artificial feeding and hydration for patients with advanced cancer who are not expected to live long. I am asked how doctors can sit back and watch while a patient starves. Relatives ask why it's such a big deal to insert a nasogastric tube, an intravenous line, or a feeding tube in the stomach to keep their loved one well for a little longer. It is easy to forget that it is not the lack of food and drink per se, but the cancer that is causing the sharp decline.

Every oncologist finds these heartfelt appeals for intervention sorrowful – they are backed by the best intentions of the family. But artificial nutrition methods are not long-term solutions in cancer management. They are uncomfortable, painful and even dangerous. For example, a nasogastric tube, inserted through the nose and entering the stomach, can cause ulceration, infection or bleeding along its journey. An intravenous (IV) line must be replaced regularly and has a high rate of becoming painfully infected. A feeding tube in the stomach can become dislodged and infected. Artificial feeding can also exacerbate bloating, pain and constipation. Moreover, these interventions don't prolong life and detract from the quality of life, in part by extending hospital stay. What's more, many patients dislike them, become fed up and ask to have them removed.

I hope you can see the sound reasons behind the majority of cancer patients with advanced cancer not being given artificial feeding and hydration. But depending on how this is communicated, the matter can become the focus of acrimonious debate between doctor and patient or carer. Patients who insist on artificial feeding often do so to placate their family, to avoid the appearance of giving up. But many patients expressly forbid artificial nutrition because they accept that it will not alter their prognosis. If you think this issue will become contentious, I recommend discussing it with your family ahead of time. It is always preferable to calmly focus on important decisions beforehand than wrangle over matters under pressure.

For patients who are able to eat and still enjoy food, it is sensible to make modest and sensible modifications to avoid problems, and I find most of my patients manage this. As one put it, 'I regret that it's a bit late, but I want to try to live a healthy life to fight this.' Some people might omit foods that provoke reflux or ones they find hard to digest. Others might limit meat because they are concerned about the harmful effects of eating excess meat. Still more might give up coffee or caffeinated soft drinks because they interfere with sleep. They may pay special attention to consuming seasonal fruits and vegetables, combining this with gentle exercise. In moderation, these are all healthy initiatives.

Unfortunately, there is a growing trend to bypass regular meals for any number of specially designed diets said to benefit cancer patients.

Examples include large quantities of fresh juices, total avoidance of things like red meat and fats, only using cooking methods like boiling or steaming, eating certain foods at certain times and many more. Some people go to more extreme means to procure exotic ingredients. They import fruits, nuts and extracts advertised widely on websites. The vast majority of cancer patients use a supplemental vitamin or mineral at some point in their illness. Sometimes this is driven by the patient and other times by well-meaning relatives. Everyone has one goal in mind – to keep the patient feeling healthy and living for as long as possible. But while the incentive is understandable, there is little evidence that an exclusion diet has any real and lasting benefit, and the unwitting omission of essential nutrients such as iron or unsaturated fats may actually cause harm. Some studies show excess folic acid and vitamins A and E to be associated with worse outcomes. Herbal supplements such as St John's wort can cause an undesirably quicker clearance of cancer drugs from the body. Other supplements can potentiate the toxicity of chemotherapy. Patients who undertake extreme diets, enemas and the like with the intent of cleansing their system often end up feeling very weak and debilitated. Even if you stop the diet, the losses can be hard to compensate.

I would counsel you not to succumb to advertisements, pressure from relatives or advice garnered over the Internet. A significant number of patients spend large amounts of money importing so-called healing foods, travelling long distances to source exclusive herbs and spices, and making a misleadingly labelled 'super-healthy lifestyle' their chief preoccupation. While they may find this an appropriate short-term focus for their energies, these pursuits are seldom rewarding in the longer term. Many patients become malnourished and disillusioned, not to mention financially bereft. 'I can't believe how I let myself be led by the glossy advertisements to spend thousands of dollars on so-called miracle foods,'one gloomily admitted to me. 'I should have known better.'

The fact that complementary and alternative health pursuits are a multi-billion-dollar industry tells us that many patients, perhaps most, dip into them at some time, whether it be a particular diet, herb or pill. It is understandable that when patients realize that chemotherapy has many limitations, and that despite major advances, many cancers still come with a poor prognosis, they look to other avenues of help. As I discussed elsewhere, always be aware that complementary and alternative health practitioners do not face the same burden of proof as those who practise conventional medicine. Consequently, exaggerated claims are easier to make and are seldom verified unless there are major and persistent complaints. Even then, regulation is lax. As with natural therapies for cancer, it is ineffective to put a blanket ban on supplements, vitamins and minerals and special diets. If you are iron-deficient through bleeding or have a condition that predisposes you to malabsorption of certain nutrients, supplements have a role. But most patients do not benefit from supplements. Since pursuits considered 'banned' by doctors automatically take on an attraction of their own, I prefer to remind patients of the saying 'Everything in moderation'. This means eating, drinking and exercising in reasonable amounts and not relying on any one agent of change. This is the least stressful arrangement not only for the patient, but also for the family who must constantly make adjustments when one member falls ill.

'But isn't it possible that you just don't know how good my imported dietary powder really is?' a patient persisted. Like her, patients often wonder why particular alternative remedies are dismissed out of hand by an oncologist who hasn't even heard of them. In my experience doctors are reacting to the unregulated way in which alternative health industries can promote their wares. In contrast, every step of medical practice is keenly watched, regulated and scrutinized for its evidence base. The rigour with which it is scrutinized keeps it accountable. If alternative therapies and miracle diets did the good they are meant to, then more people would be alive as a result.

I appreciate that an argument against alternative medicines is not a reason for having chemotherapy – we have discussed that chemotherapy is toxic and responsible for serious side effects. The difference is that there is a scientific body of evidence supporting chemotherapy and even where there is not, the potential benefits and harms can be openly discussed and monitored. You can look them up, read about them and seek a second opinion about their use. Not all, but many, side effects are predictable, preventable or manageable. This is seldom the case with the more extreme alternative medicines, whose users can end up much worse as a result.

I would urge you to not spend vast amounts of money pursuing unrealistic goals. If your cancer has progressed through multiple lines of therapy, it is unlikely that a herb, juice or enema can cure you but they could do harm. If you are unsure, talk to a doctor or nurse. They may have seen other patients take the path you are planning on and might counsel you on being prudent without dissuading you. Talk to your family about how best to spend time together, embracing the things that matter. It will hopefully help you look back with satisfaction.

Key Points

- Anxiety about appetite and diet is exceedingly common, affecting patients and their carers.
- Accept that you may not have a robust appetite, and continue to lose weight despite trying, especially if you have advanced cancer.
- Weight loss or gain is not your fault. It is a part of having cancer and is very difficult to alter.
- Regard 'miracle' and exotic nutritional products with great caution. A good diet does not have to be expensive or involved.

18

Why Natural Therapies Aren't the Answer

The reports look concerning. There was a large, bleeding cancer of the colon, which took an adept surgeon many hours to stem. The pathologist confirms what the surgeon saw, that there were many lymph glands affected and the features look aggressive.

Eddie is only thirty-eight years old. I glance again at the date of his surgery, nearly four months ago. The window of opportunity to receive chemotherapy is diminishing. Why hasn't he come to see me in all this time?

My first dismayed thought is that this is another system error, the kind that is seen a handful of times every year when a patient becomes lost in the maze of the health care network. Some patients are oblivious to the fact that they must see an oncologist after their operation. Sometimes they claim that they weren't referred, while others didn't know whom to ask when an expected appointment never arrived. 'I just thought they changed their mind, and that if it was important someone would call me,' explained one patient, who showed up to the clinic nearly two years after surgery, prompted by her GP, who had met her only after the disease had spread widely.

As I prepare to call in Eddie I wonder what his reason for non-attendance after surgery will be, but I mentally prepare myself to meet an angry patient. Of all the things I dislike, it is the knowledge that something simple in patient care went amiss – a faxed referral that never arrived, a letter mailed to the wrong address, a staff member who misjudged the importance of timing. These very human errors still occur despite sophisticated systems but when a life is endangered, they are uncomfortable to explain. The more I think about it, the more I fear Eddie's irritation will be compounded when he discovers the unnecessary delay in beginning chemotherapy.

'Hi, doc!' he greets me lightly, seemingly at ease. 'Hang on just a second.' His fingers work overtime to text a woman, who soon rushes down the corridor, balancing a phone and two herbal teas in her hands. They walk into my room together. He introduces her as his wife, Charlotte. He's a personal trainer and she a primary-school teacher.

Once they are seated, I ask him, 'How are you doing?'

'Okay,' he says. 'But obviously not great because I wouldn't be here to see you, right?'

'So you had an operation four months ago. Has your recovery been long?'

'No, no. I bounced back really quickly after the operation. I was lucky.'

'He was doing a small modelling job just seven weeks later,' adds Charlotte, explaining that most of his photo shoots involve Eddie's face, rendering his abdominal scar irrelevant.

'I didn't keep your earlier appointment because I saw someone else close to home,' Eddie continues. He lives a few hours away in a country town, and I feel instantly relieved that his care has not been compromised by our delay.

'So how is the chemo going?' I ask, expecting him to be halfway through the standard recommendation.

'I'm not having chemo. I decided against it.'

Puzzled, I ask, 'Then why are there so many IV marks on your arms?'

'I'm having intravenous nutrients and healing foods,' Eddie tells me. 'We decided on natural therapy because we don't believe in the way chemo treats your body.' Charlotte regards my incredulous expression sympathetically.

My mind immediately flies to who is advising him and how much it's costing. I am full of questions but I remind myself that every oncologist meets a patient like Eddie every year. 'Tell me more,' I say.

'As you know, the surgeon got the whole lot out. He sent me to an oncologist but I didn't like the way she talked. I went to a second oncologist who just backed up the first one, so it seemed a waste of time.'

Charlotte chips in. 'I mean, they were both really negative about natural therapy and only wanted to discuss chemotherapy. We just didn't get the right vibe.'

'So we found this natural therapist through a friend,' Eddie explains, 'and he sounded great. No offence to you, but I'm really impressed with what's out there to cure cancer.'

Another patient has recently made me aware of a new natural therapy being marketed for bowel cancer. 'Tell me what's impressive,' I prompt him.

'Everything,' Eddie enthuses. 'This guy gets good results with all kinds of cancer. I did a lot of reading about his therapy, as well as about the side effects of chemo, which run into pages. To me it was clear I wanted something natural that didn't cause any problems.'

'And why do you need them intravenously?' I try hard to keep my tone neutral.

'The IV treatment primes his body so that the rest of the treatment is more successful,' Charlotte enthuses. 'This is a specific European treatment made from exclusive, internationally sourced herbs and nutrients that most people haven't heard of.'

She sounds as if she has memorized the advertisement. I recall a colleague's recent lament. 'Each time I think I've heard it all before, someone surprises me. If it's not lavender, it's olive extract. One day it's apricot kernels, the next goji berries. One month, a diet of fruit juice is in vogue; another month it's a regimen that bans them. The dictats are no less confusing than our medical protocols.'

Eddie breaks into my thoughts. 'This guy is just really nice. He's very reassuring, seems to know what he is doing, and has hundreds of testimonials.'

I wonder why he feels such testimonials are worth more than a wealth of experience in a first-class health care system, though I realize how terribly defensive that sounds. I'm reminded that I have still no idea what Eddie is doing in my office.

'So, Eddie, how can I help you?'

'I also see a faith healer who heard you on radio. He said you were different – that you would support my needs.'

When I continue to look puzzled, Charlotte says, 'He told us that some oncologists don't favour futile medical treatments and you would support Eddie's natural therapy and faith healing.'

My spine stiffens. To a doctor, integrity of practice means everything. Every oncologist is different in some way, but to imply that I send my patients to faith healers instead of recommending chemotherapy fundamentally misconstrues my advice. In fact, I recall the radio talk, which centred on forgoing futile interventions at the end of life in favour of quality. In its aftermath, a natural healer had invited me to join the board of his newly formed company, which I declined. The company made unfounded claims about curing cancer.

'Eddie, I want to clarify that I don't even know who sent you here. And I have to tell you that I think the treatment you are having is bogus. It is not useful, potentially dangerous, probably very expensive, and I daresay you are being manipulated.'

The couple looks at each other, taken aback.

Eddie rubs his chin thoughtfully. 'So you don't believe in the body's own power to heal?'

'I actually do. I see the body doing amazing things. But I don't think that intravenous vitamins and other natural extracts have a lot to do with it. Your body excretes most of it anyway.'

'But vitamins cure cancer.'

'No, they don't. In fact, there is evidence to the contrary – that high-dose vitamins can cause harm.'

'So what would you recommend?'

'You won't like it, but I believe you should have chemotherapy, Eddie. A young man like you with an aggressive cancer is at high risk of recurrence. I would like to see you under close medical supervision.' Seeing his disappointed expression, I adopt a more conciliatory tone. 'You may not agree with the other oncologists' style, but their opinion is valid. It's based on decades of evidence from around the world. And bowel cancer is one of the more visible success stories of cancer. People are living longer thanks to better treatments and your oncologists want to ensure you don't miss out.'

'But chemotherapy upsets your internal balance whereas natural therapies restore it,' Charlotte says. 'That's what our therapist says.'

'It's true chemotherapy gives you side effects, but that statement doesn't really mean anything, Charlotte. Yes, there are patients in whom the risks of chemotherapy outweigh the benefits, but Eddie is not one of them. In fact, his case is the opposite. I think chemotherapy offers him a better long-term outcome.'

'How can you prove chemotherapy works?'

'I honestly can't,' I reply. 'There is no test except people's cumulative experience. But tell me, how do you prove natural therapies work?'

'Because they're in tune with your body,' Eddie says. Charlotte adds, 'Everyone has vitamins inside them, but Eddie just needs super doses.'

We go around the subject a bit more but their mind is made up and it's time to end the consultation.

'So, just to make sure,' I sum up, 'You are not interested in having chemotherapy and I don't need to see you again since you come from so far away too.'

'Well, we were hoping we could keep seeing an oncologist while we did *our* thing.' For the first time, Eddie's voice takes on a slightly pleading quality.

'The therapist said that Eddie will need special tests from time to time to make sure the treatment is working,' Charlotte adds. I let her finish, although I know what's coming. 'But he can't order medical tests and our family doctor refuses to help us.'

As an oncologist, I will go to great lengths to accommodate the needs of patients, but this is where I draw the line.

'I'm sorry but I can't take on that job, either. If the natural therapist claims to offer you a cure for cancer, he will also have to think of how to test you.'

Eddie's face falls. I can tell he and his wife are annoyed, and the next exchange is curt.

'So you think my natural therapy is useless.'

'I don't think that it replaces chemotherapy.'

'How can you be sure?'

'I can only be as sure as medical evidence allows me, and I agree that I can't guarantee having chemotherapy will cure you.'

'I don't buy the notion that chemotherapy is helpful at all.'

'You don't have to, Eddie, but you came here for my honest opinion and you have it.'

I reflect that for all his bravado, Eddie looks anxious and even frightened. A healthy young man, he didn't expect to be diagnosed with cancer. Nobody does. I'm sure you felt overwhelmed the first time you consulted an oncologist. After all, it takes a leap of faith to trust a stranger to safeguard your health.

I am aware that with the flourish of a pen, I can sign off on chemotherapy that can sometimes make the difference between life and death. Regarding this from a patient's perspective, this is more than enough to justify a healthy dose of scepticism about an oncologist's recommendation. I don't mind scepticism – it keeps me alert and engaged in my job, reminding me that behind every pathology report there is a human being.

As I have emphasized in previous chapters, no oncologist objects to active and engaged questioning – it actually makes our job easier. You certainly should question your doctor to ensure you understand the decisions about your health. But then remember that when you meet people who claim to match an oncologist's professional opinion, or promise better results without any toxicity, they deserve to be judged by the same high standards. Every cancer patient needs to ask why an oncologist would withhold a meaningful and life-saving therapy from a patient that a natural therapist or faith healer promises to deliver. Every cancer patient needs to ask, 'Is it too good to be true?'. Because unfortunately, as the adage goes, it probably is.

In parting, Eddie expresses his disappointment. 'I'd heard so much about you. I really thought you would be different.'

One year later, I run into a rural oncologist at a conference who mentions a recent case of a young man briefly in his care who died. The oncologist wonders whether chemotherapy would have helped him live longer and expresses his frustration that he could not convince his patient to have it. From other details, I quickly recognize Eddie and Charlotte as the subject of his story, although the oncologist doesn't know that they once sought my advice.

I learn that Eddie's disease spread to the liver. He went back to the same natural therapist, who recommended more vitamins and natural products until Eddie was too weak and malnourished to stand up without assistance. He was told there was nothing else the natural therapist could do and to seek help at the local emergency room. There were no further phone calls or correspondence from his therapist. When Eddie landed in emergency on a busy Saturday night, there was no one his doctors could call for a background report.

Eventually, Eddie was moved to a hospice where his deterioration continued. He volunteered that he had spent over $70,000 pursuing alternative therapy. In the final week of his life, moved by receiving devoted and non-judgemental care, he expressed doubt that his money had been well spent. On his death, Charlotte was unemployed and faced a large debt. She was forced to sell their house and moved in with her sister. A fraudulent promise not only proved disastrous and painful for Eddie, but also left him with a deep sense of abandonment at the end. Charlotte faces a long period of rebuilding, emotionally and financially.

I share this story with you in detail not to frighten you. If you have made up your mind to have alternative therapy for cancer, you are probably thinking that I am trying to talk you out of it. I am not. You are absolutely entitled to your own view and no oncologist will deny that chemotherapy is toxic. Much as we would like, no oncologist will guarantee that having chemotherapy will save your life. But do consider that just as things can go wrong with chemotherapy, so they can with natural therapy, which is not as safe, pure and risk-free as its proponents will tell you.

Genetic 'fingerprinting' of many popular herbal supplements, used for a range of illnesses including cancer, reveals that as many as half are simply not what they claim. In other words, natural elements are diluted, adulterated or sometimes, replaced entirely by cheap fillers like soy and wheat. If you have a nut allergy, a trace of nut filler may be all you need to trigger a deadly anaphylaxis. Some replacements can be toxic to humans or interfere with prescription medication. The problem with the supplement and alternative medicine industry is that it is unregulated. You cannot be sure that you are taking what you think you are. Prescription drugs must be rigorously scrutinized and assessed before being made widely available – and even then, unforeseen problems occur. But vitamin and all manner of supplements are considered safe unless proven otherwise and products are removed from shelves only after numerous complaints, and then too, there is no rigorous oversight of the process.

I accept as an oncologist that many, if not most, of my patients use herbal supplements and alternative medicines – after all, this is a flourishing multi-billion-dollar industry and it's naive to assume otherwise. I would encourage you to discuss such use with your oncologist. Sometimes, your oncologist's advice may help you avoid a harmful drug interaction. Other times, it is a signal of trust in your oncologist to let her into your decisions.

Here, I should distinguish between complementary therapy such as yoga, meditation and mindfulness activities and alternative therapy consisting of unproven remedies. Almost every oncologist acknowledges the importance of tending to the mind-body axis as part of comprehensive cancer treatment. It is when the treatment strays into elimination diets, super foods and vitamin megadoses that oncologists become wary.

'I am tired of everyone being negative about alternative therapy,' a patient grumbled.

I understand the patient's complaint. After all, the theme of this book is about having control and exerting choice. You can choose to forego chemotherapy or other conventional treatments, and you can certainly choose an alternative path of care. But every oncologist you meet who seems to be against your wishes is probably striving to serve your best interest. It is ultimately for you to decide.

Key Points

- You will almost certainly encounter natural therapies and alternative medicine that promise to cure cancer.
- Complementary therapies such as yoga, meditation and mindfulness can assist with symptoms but interventions or products that make exaggerated claims of benefit should be regarded with caution.
- Some alternative therapies are harmful and may interfere with chemotherapy; be open with your oncologist if you are taking any.
- Alternative therapies can be costly and leave patients and their families with large debts without any benefit to disease.

19

How Much Exercise Should I Be Doing?

'Try to get some exercise,' I suggested to Edward, a man in his sixties who was receiving chemotherapy and complained of incessant fatigue. His days were either spent battling nausea or combating sleepiness and he was frustrated that someone formerly as fit as him had seen such a quick decline in his condition. He used to enjoy getting out and about in his vintage car, but hadn't left his house for days and was becoming irritable with his wife.

He looked at me as if I was mad. 'Did you hear me, doc? I'm so tired that I can't be bothered buttering my bread – and you want me to drive!'

'Maybe not driving, but how about a walk in the park, as you used to enjoy so much?'

'I couldn't – I'd collapse midway.'

'You might be surprised,' I said. 'You were playing squash twice a week before you got sick.'

Fed up with being tired, Edward reluctantly agreed to give gentle exercise a try. 'I'll try anything, although what you're saying seems counter-intuitive to me.'

We worked out a very modest exercise plan. It involved walking fifteen minutes from his house to the park with his wife on three days of the week. His son agreed to drive behind him in case he really felt he needed a ride back. Edward felt disappointed at the miserly goal and regretted that he would never regain his former fitness.

The first day he got dressed, his sports shoes didn't fit his swollen legs, but he found his son's larger pair and went out with his wife holding his hand all the way to steady him. The walk took Edward thirty minutes and he felt exhausted, but for the last five minutes he managed to walk without support. Too tired to contemplate returning home, he sat down on a bench and watched some local children play in the park. His son drove him back and he spent the rest of the day sleeping. Two days later he felt ready to do it again. This time, he let go of his wife's hand for ten minutes and finished the walk in less time. Again, he sat on the bench. His wife brought out some snacks and they sat together in the sunshine. This time, they met a neighbour who was delighted to see him after months. Talking to him made Edward realize how much he had missed the company of his neighbours and friends, whom they used to see regularly before he fell ill.

That weekend there was a note in their mailbox from a friend. 'Eddie, I am recovering from a hip operation. Would you like a very slow companion on some of your walks?' Eddie couldn't believe how happy he was to hear from his old squash friend. Before he knew it, he was walking four days a week with a different person each time. The walks still took longer than he liked and he could only do them one way, but at our next appointment he seemed much brighter. 'I didn't realize how isolated I'd become. Simply being outside and watching others rejuvenates me. I also forget my problems when I am walking.'

In another month, Edward had built up to walking every day, regaining some friends along the way. He was less irritable, a little less tired, and more optimistic about his future. When he finished chemotherapy he continued to set himself small, incremental goals. It took him three years to return to playing squash. I asked him what the greatest obstacle to exercise during chemotherapy had been. He replied that it was the assumption that exercise was all or nothing. 'I thought that if I couldn't play high-intensity sport, there was no point in doing a few laps of the streets because it just wasn't enough exercise. It took me a while to appreciate that even the minor exercise I was doing made a difference and then I could reset my expectations. For me, that was the best recovery tool.'

A second patient called Alia comes to mind. Alia was an Arabic patient who had never exercised in her life. After finishing chemotherapy for breast cancer she found herself having gained significant weight.

She started a diet but her hormonal therapy caused so much joint pain that she couldn't walk easily. She complained that at the age of forty-five she found herself unable to fit into any of her old clothes and felt like 'an old lady with rheumatism'. Alia's doctor prescribed antidepressants, which caused further weight gain and insomnia, and in turn made her tired during the day. She also developed high blood pressure and when I saw her for a follow-up appointment she said morosely that although she was taking more pills, she felt worse. 'My daughter is a fitness instructor and she says I need exercise, but I can't do anything.'

I suggested that one thing Alia hadn't tried was the hydrotherapy pool, something that had helped other patients like her. The poor lady balked at the very thought of putting on a swimming costume and swimming in mixed-gender pools. 'I'm sorry but this would be too embarrassing for me. I couldn't dress like that in public.' Eventually, with her daughter's encouragement, she found a costume that provided adequate cover. She wore it at home for a week to get over her reservations before going to the pool early one morning when few people were around. Then, along with her daughter, she literally took the plunge. Alia walked the length of the pool and found herself soothed by the warm water. To her pleasant surprise she met other people who couldn't swim but used the pool for exercise. A few weeks later, her daughter coaxed her into trying a weights class held in the pool. Over four months, Alia lost weight, regained muscle tone and felt much better psychologically. She no longer needed her sleeping tablet or blood pressure medication and talked to her doctor about stopping her antidepressants. She found it hard to believe the difference that exercise had made to her life and felt very grateful for being persuaded to try the pool.

Cancer and its treatment are associated with a number of serious physical and psychological symptoms. Exercise is widely believed to improve these symptoms. Studies of exercise during and after cancer treatment show a consistent trend towards improvement in the lives of patients.

There are different kinds of exercise that you might find helpful. Aerobic exercise includes walking, cycling, jogging and swimming, which increase your heart rate. Resistance exercises refer to the use of free or fixed weights that help you build muscle strength, tone and endurance. Relaxation exercises include yoga, t'ai chi and other types of mindfulness practice. The benefits of exercise include healthy weight maintenance, improved functional capacity and increased muscle strength. And while it can often be hard to measure these things objectively, cancer patients do report a number of psychological benefits, including improvements in anxiety, fatigue, self-esteem, depression, sleep quality and overall quality of life.

Patients who are encouraged by their doctor to participate in some form of exercise are more likely to adopt a formal programme, but like Alia and Edward, you may feel so overwhelmed by your condition that exercise is the last thing on your mind. Like many patients, you might fear that exercise could waste your small and precious reserve of energy, which you need to fight your illness. Or perhaps exercise sounds like yet another unwelcome prescription in your overloaded life.

The first thing I would say is that there is no fixed prescription for exercise. From the type of exercise to the amount undertaken, it will depend on what you like to do and what your body is capable of. You may decide to continue your previous preferred forms of exercise but reduce the intensity. Some patients are too tired in the initial days after chemotherapy but feel well enough in the intervening time before the next cycle to get out. Others do some exercise on most days but keep it gentle; for example, a short stroll instead of a run, or a brief time on the bike or in the swimming pool. You may exchange heavy weights for lighter ones or prefer to potter in the yard as you always have.

Body image and what others might think about possibly altered looks, such as the loss of hair associated with chemo, can figure on many patients' minds. If you have gained weight during cancer treatment, it may be prudent to combine exercise with a sensibly controlled diet. Chemotherapy drugs and the steroids that often accompany them cause undesirable weight gain in many patients. As studies demonstrate that being overweight is related to an increased risk of cancer recurrence, it pays to be attentive to diet and exercise. Discuss it with your oncologist. If your oncologist doesn't have the time or capacity to advise you in detail, find someone else.

If you have advanced cancer, your challenge is usually to preserve muscle mass and weight. Then, if you can tolerate them, you may wish to combine protein-rich food and high-calorie supplements with gentle aerobic or strength-based exercises, which promote mobility, function and quality of life. Combining active exercise with meditation, yoga or t'ai chi is useful without being fatigued. Chances are that the better you feel about yourself the more likely you are to adhere to healthy living habits.

Some patients express doubt in their ability to get into a routine of exercise and feel as if they need a personal trainer or a structured programme, with a cost they cannot afford. If there is a specific issue or a pre-existing injury that concerns you, consult a physiotherapist, gym instructor or other expert. But in most instances you don't need them. Begin gently and do what your body allows. Don't have unrealistic expectations and don't feel let down if at first you find it hard. Focus on some of the gains in quality of life that may be in store for you, whether they are catching up with an old friend for a stroll, seeing the sun filter through the trees, or feeling more rested and less anxious. As they say, don't just sit there, do something!

I often meet patients who give up on the prospect of exercising and go into a form of hibernation. But when they pull themselves out of this state, they feel proud and reinvigorated. Amongst my own patients, I see a lady who has breast cancer involving her bones. Despite having pain in her hips, for which she has received radiation therapy, she has never stopped dancing. She says that dancing with her husband is her lifeblood and I see how it sustains her spirits. Another patient with advanced lung cancer has dramatically reduced his exercise but still goes out every day with his oxygen cylinder tucked inside his walking frame. He says that even the short time of being outside the house makes him feel part of the world.

So I hope I have demonstrated that there is no one proven way to exercise and it is certainly not meant to be a chore. Exercise has a wide range of health benefits. You have nothing to lose, so give it a try.

Key Points

- Exercise is important for physical and emotional health. Gentle exercise can increase feelings of wellness and aid recovery.
- Be prepared to moderate your expectations of exercise but don't assume it has to be all or nothing. Start or resume slowly and work up to a safe and comfortable level.
- There is no need for an expensive or involved exercise programme; common-sense measures work.

20

I'm Always Tired

If we could find a way of banishing fatigue in cancer we would all be winners. It is the rare patient with cancer who doesn't feel tired and even those with a strong constitution observe how fatigue weighs on their days. 'I can't believe how tired I feel all the time,' is a common refrain heard from patients. 'It's the worst part of having chemotherapy.' A patient recently told me that she found herself unable to summon the energy to talk when she was undergoing chemotherapy. Now recovered, she still feels incredulous when recalling the experience.

You might belong anywhere along the spectrum of tiredness – for some, it is a nuisance that they manage to get around, but for many others it is debilitating. Many people can't understand how they can go from someone who used to be very fit to not having the energy to walk around the house or engage in conversation. One woman told me that after every chemotherapy cycle she took to her bed for the next ten days. 'Each time I felt I wouldn't be able to get up, but miraculously, I did.'

Whereas modern treatment methods successfully address troublesome symptoms such as nausea, pain or insomnia in many if not all patients, a good remedy for fatigue has been elusive. The average person feels tired after a long run, a busy day at the office or a session of moving heavy furniture. Tiredness of this sort improves with food and drink, a long shower or a restful sleep. I daresay the tiredness even feels good. It is well known that exercise induces hormones that induce a sense of achievement and well-being.

But if you are a cancer patient, you know that your tiredness is far from exhilarating. Cancer fatigue is a persistent, pervasive feeling of exhaustion that is disproportionate to your level of activity and interferes with daily life. It seems unresponsive to the usual steps to relieve it and impacts personal and professional relationships, employment and social activities. Fatigue is especially prominent amongst patients undergoing chemotherapy and those with advanced cancer, but almost everyone affected by cancer feels it in some way. People describe being fed up of the unshakeable feeling that prevents them from doing enjoyable things. 'It's like "I can't be bothered" endlessly multiplied and with no end in sight,' a lady receiving chemotherapy told me. Another man with advanced prostate cancer said, 'I don't expect miracles, but it would be so nice to have the energy to sit outside.'

Unlike a broken arm or a bandaged wound, an invisible feeling like fatigue is hard to convey, especially if you otherwise appear in reasonable physical shape. It is also difficult to grade or quantify – how you judge it depends on many factors, not all of which are under an individual's control. The human body undergoes numerous hormonal, emotional and neural changes during cancer. But while the details of these changes are complex, there is no doubt that fatigue adds to the burden of suffering.

Patients are often hard on themselves. When I ask about fatigue, they sometimes say, 'I just can't get myself going – I know, I'm probably being lazy.' But it's not just laziness, cancer fatigue is real. Far too many people battle cancer fatigue but feel reluctant to say so due to fears of how others will judge them. For some, keeping up the appearance of being strong and stoic is important. A young mother couldn't bring herself to tell her children that she felt tired, so she kept pushing herself to do activities that she privately admitted she could barely keep up with. A retired farmer didn't want his wife to mention selling their farm, so he kept going out to milk the cows although he then had to spend the afternoon in bed. If you are on chemotherapy you might conceal the full extent of your fatigue from your oncologist for fear of treatment being stopped. You might downplay fatigue to avoid disappointing loved ones or visitors who have taken the trouble to come from far. While these feelings are understandable, it is vital that you discuss your fatigue with your doctor or nurse. Persistent fatigue is a reliable indication of how you are faring on treatment. Far from hampering your treatment plan, admitting fatigue sends an important signal to your oncologist to modify things, especially by curbing toxic treatments that are contributing to the symptom.

There are a few important things you can explore with your oncologist if you are concerned by tiredness. The first thing to ask is whether your treatment itself is contributing to fatigue. Doctors rate chemotherapies from mild to aggressive and patients from robust to frail, but we know that we still can't accurately predict how someone will handle chemotherapy. I have seen a ninety-year-old man sail through chemotherapy that put a sixty-year-old in hospital. So the first thing is to not be entirely swayed by descriptions of how a particular chemotherapy is *supposed* to affect you. Each of a dozen patients on the same regimen may experience different toxicities. For some, nausea will prevail over nerve problems. Some will be troubled by infections or diarrhoea. For others, fatigue will be the deal-breaker. Oncologists can broadly predict toxicities, but unfortunately, predicting their severity in an individual is not an exact science. So when your oncologist mentions a chance of infection it isn't easy to say whether it will be a minor setback or a full-blown pneumonia resulting in admission to an intensive care unit.

I suggest using descriptive examples of your fatigue when talking to your doctor, to provide some context. Instead of just saying 'I feel ragged' say, 'I've vacuumed my house all of my life but now I get tired after five minutes.' Or, 'Up until last month, I could climb the stairs at home but now I stay downstairs.' 'I have always been an active golfer but now I'm too tired to pick up the club.' Sometimes fatigue becomes such a part of the new you that it's hard to explain it to others. 'I'm so used to feeling tired that I can't remember what it was like to be well,' someone said. At these times it can be useful to note what a family member or friend observes about you. 'My son came home the other day and commented that the effort of sitting down to dinner made me tired. He said I was different two weeks ago.'

Fatigue is not always reflected in your blood tests, unless you are anaemic or have an obvious organ dysfunction. It's a misconception that as long as your blood tests are alright nothing needs to change with your chemotherapy. Your level of fatigue – and hence the ability to do things – is a much better indicator of your welfare than a set of blood tests. Acknowledging your fatigue to yourself and mentioning it to your oncologist is a good start to managing it.

One response to your fatigue may be to reduce, defer or stop chemotherapy to see if this allays the problem. One of the commonest fears people express is that stopping chemotherapy will fuel cancer growth. You may be genuinely afraid that by complaining excessively about tiredness you will short-change yourself of useful treatment. While this is a reasonable concern, it isn't valid in many situations. Sometimes reducing the dose or deferring a cycle of chemotherapy is the best way to ensure long-term treatment, because you allow your body to recover more completely between cycles. Many types of chemotherapy are calculated based on your height and weight, but it's conceivable that the initial dose of chemotherapy is toxic for you, in which case the dose needs to be reduced quickly before problems mount.

Not uncommonly, overwhelming fatigue is accompanied by other symptoms such as nausea, anorexia, diarrhoea or pain. Modifying the chemotherapy dose may ease these other side effects. If no amount of drug adjustment helps, the more important question to ask is whether the ongoing toxicities justify the treatment, as we discussed in earlier chapters. What is the ultimate benefit to you from putting up with the side effects? For therapy given with curative intent for a defined period, the answer may be that it's worth pushing on – this too depending on your age, other illnesses and your personal philosophy. But when the treatment is palliative – that is, non-curative, where the benefits can be far more modest – it is important to appraise your situation realistically.

Whatever the case, if you are so tired from your treatment that you spend most of the intervening time in bed recovering from it or dreading returning for more, you should talk to your oncologist. Try to not let the problem get to an unmanageable point before mentioning your concern. 'I thought you could tell how bad I felt,' a patient once protested after he landed in hospital. Many patients feel that their discomfort is written on their face, or their true feelings about chemotherapy are interwoven amongst what they actually say, but you should never rely on doctors and nurses to read between the lines when it comes to your health. Openly mention the things that trouble you.

Just because you have cancer doesn't mean that your fatigue is solely as a result of cancer. Your oncologist should still search for correctable causes like anaemia, thyroid conditions, malnutrition, pain, worsening of pre-existing or coexisting chronic disease like heart or kidney failure and insomnia. Correctly identified, their management can ameliorate, if not entirely dispel, fatigue. This is another reason to be open with your oncologist.

Another common cause of fatigue is depression, which requires specialized attention. Depression is widely prevalent amongst cancer patients and studies estimate that up to a third of cancer patients suffer from it, although the figure could well be higher. Moreover, nearly half of these patients are not treated due to under-recognition, as well as the belief that it is 'natural' to be depressed in the circumstances. This belief is untrue. While it's conceivable that almost every cancer patient feels disheartened or sad from time to time, depression is a pervasive emotional state that affects many aspects of daily life, from nutrition and sleep to self-image and relationships with others. Depression is a manageable illness, provided it can be identified and dealt with. Depression may be associated with prolonged and difficult chemotherapy courses, multiple concurrent illnesses, poor social supports, missing emotional and spiritual care or a previous history of mood disorders. Of course, not everyone who is depressed may have these factors and not everyone who ticks these boxes will become depressed, but it's helpful to recognize some of the important risk factors for depression and ask for help.

Your oncologist will spend most of your consultations dealing directly with cancer treatment and its complications – this is necessary, but might leave important issues in your life untouched. Oncologists aren't trained in the intricacies of depression diagnosis and management and many will confess to an inability to recognize it in the busy run of their day. They can, however, refer you to an appropriate source for help, ranging from specialized nurses and support groups to psychologists and psychiatrists.

Again, many patients are reticent to even mention depression to their oncologist for fear of it affecting their medical treatment, but effective side-by-side management of depression and cancer is possible, and indeed, important for best results. If you think that you are experiencing more than the usual occasional episode of feeling anxious, sad or hopeless, mention this to your doctor and discuss a formal assessment. An assessment will yield some answers to inform one of a number of treatments, or it may clear the air and reassure both you and your doctor that your fatigue has an explanation other than depression.

You might be so occupied by chemotherapy or other medical commitments that you are loath to take on another appointment to explore your psychological health. But taking care of your mind is vital to dealing with the journey of cancer.

Successful identification and abatement of depression takes weeks to months. Poor mental health can deeply affect your entire experience of cancer and jeopardize treatment, but if depression is treated, it may help you to adhere to useful therapy. In such cases, it is important to remember that depression is not only your problem but also your family's, because of the way depression affects family dynamics.

So, physical fitness and emotional well-being are important aspects of managing fatigue. As discussed in the previous chapter, even the most devoted and health-conscious patients can let exercise lapse from their daily activities as they become preoccupied by the new world of cancer. But we are increasingly realizing the vital role that exercise plays in cancer.

I hope you now understand that there are many reasons why you might be fatigued. Unfortunately, even when all of the things we have discussed are addressed, there will be some patients who remain overwhelmed by fatigue. Since the depth of such fatigue is invisible, it is easy for onlookers to be frustrated by your inability to be active and engaged. But in fact, it is the rare patient who just wants to rest all the time. So if you are feeling like this, remember that it is not your fault. Your fatigue is a manifestation of the profound effect of cancer on physical and emotional well-being. People who are facing this degree of fatigue temporarily need our support in looking to a more active future. Those who are more seriously ill also need our emotional support and backing to spend their remaining days comfortably. (Of course, for those who are cured of cancer or in remission, emotional support is no less important as they continue with life.) You may benefit from the quiet presence of family and reassurance that it is okay to feel the way you do. If you are a carer, you can encourage alertness through short conversations, craft, recording memories, writing a journal or creating a legacy in some way. Listening to music or being read to can be quietly therapeutic for a patient. There may be periods of the day when you feel more like engaging – look out for the window of opportunity. Unremitting fatigue can occur in the last stages of illness, in which case palliative care may be appropriate. But being tired doesn't mean losing control of the direction of your care.

Key Points

- Tiredness is exceedingly common in cancer. For it to be effectively understood by your doctors, list the things you can no longer do.
- Fatigue can be caused by cancer treatment such as chemotherapy and prescription drugs, but this may not be the sole cause of your tiredness. Other factors such as insomnia, thyroid and mood disorders can play a role. All can be addressed.
- Gentle exercise and a healthy diet could be the antidote to your tiredness.
- Tiredness at the end of life needs recognition, emotional support and permission to rest.

21

Lost Sexuality

'How are things?' I recently asked an eighty-year-old sprightly lady having cancer treatment.

'Great,' she replied. 'Except my sex life is non-existent.'

My pen froze and for a few seconds, I didn't know where to look.

When I finally made eye contact with her again, she said, 'Seriously, this treatment has destroyed my desire, but that's okay, I can live with that. I just thought I would tell you.'

I told myself that I was having one of those slightly awkward days. The previous patient had been a woman in her fifties. By the time she came to my attention she had lost a lot of weight and spent a month in hospital. She started chemotherapy cautiously and was elated by the pleasing initial response. She attended every appointment with a lovely daughter who patiently tolerated the inevitable delays. Her mum had long accepted that she had a terminal disease with a limited prognosis and regarded every day with admirable goodwill. Just as we were finishing a consultation, she said without preface, 'And doctor, the most important question: can I have sex after chemotherapy or should I wait for a few days?'

I must confess that I nearly fell out of my chair. My first reaction was one of wonder that she even felt inclined to think about sex. She was frequently in the clutches of nausea and pain and rued the way her body looked due to excessive weight loss. I thought perhaps she was asking a hypothetical question but she put this to rest.

'I know I don't have long but I want to be happy and keep my husband happy. Sex makes us forget everything else for a while.'

I shot a glance at her daughter whose expression would have been no different were we discussing the falling rain outside. She nodded and smiled encouragingly at her mother. I realized that mother and daughter had discussed this before. I was the only person in the room who was taken aback and, frankly, embarrassed by the question, and it should have been my job to address it.

So belatedly, I told her that she could ask me all she wanted to know about sex. As we discussed lubricants and condoms, I couldn't help thinking that not once in all these years had I engaged in such an open discussion. There isn't much that is taboo in an oncologist's office – from bowel movements to menstrual periods and frequency of urination to the contents of a vomit – but sex is still a sacrosanct matter, often considered too delicate and too awkward for either doctor or patient to broach. I couldn't recall any patient more naturally inquiring than this lady. But I also couldn't remember a time that I had offered to talk about sex.

Later, I kept thinking about the joyful expression on my patient's face when she learned that having sex during cancer treatment was okay. When her daughter added that it would be emotionally therapeutic for her parents and I agreed, the patient nearly burst into tears. 'I feel I've reclaimed this last bit of joy in my life,' she declared. 'I only wish I hadn't waited so long to ask.'

The lessons fresh in my mind, I saw another lady two weeks later. She was much younger, receiving hormonal therapy for breast cancer. I couldn't help noticing that each visit saw her becoming increasingly grumpy and I gently tried to find out why. She related a host of side effects from her tablet, blaming it for her 'foggy' brain, aches and pains, heartburn, insomnia and lowered moods. 'Is the tablet affecting your sex life?' I asked casually, feeling conscious that I was prying into her personal life.

She leaped at me when she heard this. 'My sex life! Thank God, someone is finally asking! Doctor, my sex life has vanished. I used to have a healthy appetite for sex and all of a sudden I couldn't bear the thought of it. But I enjoyed sex and I now I miss it.' Again, I was taken aback by the intensity of the patient's feelings about sex. 'I don't mean to sound ungrateful', she continued, 'but if the cure for cancer ruins my sex life, I'd be quite upset.' Her problem disclosed, she expressed a keenness to solve it with a counsellor. It took her a few months to work things out, but at her next visit she reported making small but confident gains in intimacy, saying that they made her feel more complete. 'My husband says this help came too late.' Once again, I was reminded of the chasm between the assumptions that doctors and patients make about sexual needs. It also had me wondering that if women, who are generally more expressive, are reluctant to talk about it, what of male patients? They must find it impossible, or perhaps inappropriate, to discuss sex with a doctor, especially if she is a woman?

Sexuality is more than the act of intercourse – it defines how we perceive our body image, our attractiveness and attraction to a partner, and our ability to relax and enjoy sexual relations. For such an important aspect of human life, sexuality appears to be almost universally absent from conversations with cancer patients. Fatigue, pain, inattention, irritability and a myriad of other concerns manage to weave their way into discussions, but rarely sexuality. It is as if the many well-known effects of cancer on sexuality are relegated to textbooks with no relevance to the daily life of patients and their partners. Alas, this is far from true. Sexuality is deeply affected and often permanently altered by cancer treatment and the fact that we don't discuss it is a reflection of the hang-ups and misconceptions endured by both doctors and patients.

One of the key reasons that it goes unrecognized, and hence untreated, is that doctors are typically poorly trained in the facts about sexual dysfunction from cancer treatment. I cannot recall any formal education in the area and my knowledge has subsequently been gained from reading about it when faced with the occasional patient who openly mentioned the topic. Inadequate training leads to a lack of confidence in discussing the subject capably or with enough objectivity.

Patients are rarely alerted to the fact that sexual dysfunction might occur as a result of cancer treatment, and then, almost never to its true extent. They regularly find themselves confronted with a list of adversities brought about by their chosen mode of treatment – from the risk of dying during surgery from a general anaesthetic, to the potential for infections from reduced immunity. They might be told at length about the chance of heart failure, nerve damage, infertility or a second cancer resulting from treatment, and the myriad potential side effects of radiation. But the matter of altered or damaged sexuality is omitted, as if it is an unspoken but understood consequence of treatment.

Reduced libido and sexual dysfunction are exceedingly common after treatment for cancer, whether radiation, chemotherapy, surgery or hormonal therapy. Treatment can affect patients' physical, emotional or physiological functioning, with any of these leading to problems. Some problems are short-term but many persist for years or even a lifetime, causing considerable distress without the prospect of resolution if no one talks about it. The cultural and social context in which a patient regards his or her sexuality can play an important role in the delay in identification and management.

If you find yourself experiencing difficulty with intimacy and your sexual life, you might be too ready to consign the problem to the growing list of 'cancer does this' problems. This expectation means that low libido or sexual dysfunction might not seem out of place, and even if it does, it's perhaps not something to mention to your doctor. Patients fear sounding self-indulgent or worried about an 'optional extra' like sex when their very life is threatened by disease. You might be simply too embarrassed to mention sex openly for fear of embarrassing yourself and your doctor. 'I keep thinking that I can't mention sex in the same breath as my chance of recurrence to the oncologist. He would never look at me the same way again.' People also wonder what any doctor can do for such a deeply private problem and, consequently, patients end up hiding their true feelings and suffering in silence.

If a person is single, widowed or elderly, or has advanced cancer, there might be a ready assumption that a sexual relationship is not relevant. 'Don't worry about the colostomy bag,' a young woman was told by her surgeon. 'You won't be getting pregnant soon.' This woman was so mortified that she didn't have the courage to raise the matter again for a long time. To conflate sex with pregnancy, or to dismiss it as unimportant once you have cancer, is, of course, very wrong.

I imagine also that for some patients, while many symptoms lend themselves to a more obvious explanation, such as a result of chemotherapy, sexual difficulties might seem to reflect more of a personal failing. 'Maybe it's my poor attitude to any kind of intimacy these days,' a man bemoaned to me once. 'I should try harder.'

Sexual dysfunction as a result of cancer treatment affects men and women. Abdominal surgery and pelvic radiotherapy can disrupt the pelvic nerves, for example, leading to problems with sexual arousal, lubrication and ejaculation. The presence of a *stoma* – a permanent catheter or stent – can be uncomfortable, or lead to heightened consciousness about disfigurement, which in turn affects libido. A majority of men complain of some form of altered sexual function after radical prostate surgery, which is well known to cause erectile dysfunction. Testosterone-blocking therapy for prostate cancer causes hot flushes, loss of libido and changes in penile structure and function in many men. Women who undergo surgery for gynaecological cancers may also suffer from painful intercourse, lack of lubrication and lost libido. Breast cancer patients who are on hormonal therapy can experience menopausal symptoms like hot flushes, altered libido and emotional upheaval, leading to sexual difficulties. A man who developed breast cancer was too ashamed to consider sex again. Treatment-related factors such as hair loss, weight gain, mood changes and fatigue in particular, are commonly identified by patients as other barriers to having a healthy sexual life. Many patients and their partners avoid sexual intercourse because they are wary of hurting the patient or causing infections during a period of reduced immune function, or they don't think sex is appropriate during a life-threatening illness.

Awkward as it is, don't be dissuaded from discussing these and finding help from the right source. Time may restore normality but there are several aspects of sexual dysfunction that can be actively addressed. Advice on appropriate lubricants, building pelvic floor capacity, adjusting hormonal therapies and exploring non-drug measures may be all the help you need. Men may benefit from drugs to sustain an erection, penile implants, manipulation of hormonal therapy and other lifestyle measures. Openly addressing social or cultural taboos around sex as a cancer patient may be important in restoring libido for some while for others simply dismantling myths about sex and illness is important.

Whether you have a sexual difficulty, or merely a curiosity about what to expect, the key is not to be shy or assume that it is normal to have a problem, because this can lead to shame, frustration and further isolation. Do mention it to your doctor. If your doctor doesn't have the answers, which is quite possible, he or she can refer you to a sexual counsellor, endocrinologist or gynaecologist as needed.

Of course, it is also possible that your changed sexual circumstances don't bother you or your partner. Some patients describe reaching a new understanding with their partner when they are diagnosed with cancer – companionship becomes more important than sex. 'After both of our experiences with cancer, my husband and I are just content to be alive and together at the dinner table. Sex became too difficult, but we are happier than ever.'

Set your own expectations. What matters is that you feel comfortable with the level of emotional and physical intimacy in your relationship. Remember that the most common reason why low libido and sexual dysfunction is not treated is that no one wants to acknowledge it. Knowing what you do now, you should realize that it doesn't have to be so.

Key Points

- Diminished libido and sexual dysfunction are very common but usually under-treated.
- Awkward as it is, overcome your hesitation to seek advice.
- There are many modern means of addressing sexual difficulties. Your oncologist can direct you to the right professional to help you.
- It's okay if sexual changes do not trouble you and your partner. Many relationships grow stronger despite the absence of sex.

22

Tackling Anxiety and Depression

Vella was diagnosed with breast cancer at the young age of thirty. She was pregnant with her first child when the biopsy revealed an aggressive form of cancer. Since the drugs she needed were toxic to the developing fetus, she underwent a termination of pregnancy followed by a mastectomy because she felt 'betrayed' by the breast. An infection and then a clot in her leg, both fortunately improving quickly with treatment, complicated the mastectomy. On the eve of her discharge, she tripped over the bedside and fractured her foot. Luckily, she avoided surgery but was uncomfortable for weeks and couldn't drive.

As soon as she was well enough, Vella started chemotherapy. Although she had expected her treatment to be gruelling, to her pleasant surprise she did not encounter any significant side effects. She had none of the vomiting that the nurses had warned her about, her nausea was no worse than morning sickness and she didn't mind the hair loss as much as she had thought. She dealt with the fatigue better than she thought. Although she felt well to drive herself, her healing foot meant that others took turns to transport her to her many appointments. She formed even closer relationships with these people during this time.

The chemotherapy finished uneventfully and Vella was advised that she would now enter a period of close surveillance. She started attending clinic every three months, where she received a thorough check. Vella was always in good spirits, grateful to have emerged from treatment unscathed and with good support around her. She expressed great relief at her next normal mammogram.

It wasn't until the first anniversary of her diagnosis that things changed. Suddenly, she began to describe palpitations at the thought of seeing the oncologist and an inability to sleep for weeks leading up to her routine appointments. She became very fearful of the cancer returning and began to regard even the smallest symptom as being indicative of recurrence. Her colleagues at work noticed the change, as did her family. She was irritable and distracted with them but constantly apologized because she herself recognized the reactions as unusual. That year, Vella went from being a well-adjusted young woman to a self-confessed 'wreck'.

When I asked her what changed, she said that the enormity of her diagnosis had finally sunk in. 'I know it's been a whole year,' she explained apologetically, 'but it's only now that I am realizing the full extent of what happened. I got cancer, lost a child, broke a foot, missed a promotion at work and those were just the big things. There was so much else that changed in my life that now I cry at the mere thought of it.' Sympathetically, I asked whether something had happened recently to trigger her anxieties. Had a friend or family member been diagnosed with cancer? Had she read a concerning report in the newspaper? But she explained that nothing new had happened. Ironically, it was the absence of any new event in her life that had allowed her to reflect on her ordeal. 'When you are diagnosed, you are thrown into a sea of confusion, and you spend all your energy staying afloat. I had so many things to deal with at the time that I had to stay strong to get through. I also forced myself to focus on the essential things, such as eating enough to stabilize my weight or being gentle when washing around the mastectomy scar. Returning one kind phone call from work was a two-day task because I wanted to sound strong and keen to work again.'

As I nodded, she continued, 'It's only now that I recall how serious they said the cancer was, how the termination happened so fast, and how much I dreaded chemotherapy, although I was fine through it. But now, I feel lost and also lonely without a child who would have been here today. I am not the same person I was – I find myself anxious, sometimes irritable and just impatient with myself and others.' I had recommended to Vella on a previous occasion that she should see a psychiatrist but she was reluctant. 'I am not a psychiatric patient', she said. 'I am going to get over this myself.' But when I suggested it again, she seemed willing and even grateful for the offer. 'I thought I'd shake it off, but it took time to realize this is serious.'

Vella identified two issues after seeing a psychiatrist. She understood that CT scans were not a recommended part of the follow-up for her breast cancer, but she wanted to have one anyway and was too afraid to ask. This made her feel helpless. While she was correct that oncologists avoid CT scans in a range of otherwise healthy cancer patients because of the risk of unnecessary radiation exposure as well as the limited value of findings, I could see that in her case the extra reassurance was paramount. She had a CT whose normal report consoled her no end. She never asked for a repeat scan.

Her second worry related to pregnancy. She had been advised to wait for a few years but she found the thought of remaining childless daunting. We discussed that while the risk of cancer recurrence was indeed higher in the first few years there was no promise that waiting two or three years would guarantee lifelong freedom from cancer. She understood that medical advice was a guideline but she was free to follow her own instincts. To her, 'permission' from her doctors mattered greatly. She became pregnant after two-and-a-half years of follow-up and gave birth to healthy twin girls. She saw the psychiatrist only twice and has gone on to enjoy a full life. She says that her children altered her entire outlook on life, and jokes that she has no time to fret.

Wilhelm's story was different. He was diagnosed with cancer at fifty years of age when his printing business was at its peak. His family doctor organized a scan after hearing of his severe headaches over the past two months. When the scan revealed a brain tumour, Wilhelm had to be recalled from a business trip, losing an important deal in the process. He underwent a successful operation to remove the brain tumour and his neurosurgeon was happy with the results. Since the majority of brain metastases arise as a result of cancer having travelled from another organ, the so-called primary, Wilhelm had detailed tests but they were all clear. He was advised that there was a possibility that the primary cancer might eventually declare itself but it was impossible to predict when. He should return to his normal activities but stay under close surveillance. Wilhelm had been floored from the very moment he heard his diagnosis. No amount of reassurance or discussion of the available evidence changed his initial reaction of complete shock. So, this is how he interpreted the advice about surveillance. 'They are just waiting for another cancer to come up, and that will be the end of me.' When his wife tried to point out the positive news that he was free of cancer, he bitterly told her that she didn't understand. He repeated that he couldn't fathom his stress headaches had meant anything more. His family watched helplessly as the initial anxiety and depression never gave way to his former self. Two years passed and there was no sign of cancer, but Wilhelm believed that he was merely waiting to die. He became disinterested in his business and eventually sold it to his partners. Although they paid him a handsome price for his share, he perceived the affair as a loss. He stopped seeing his friends to 'protect them from my grief'. Five years on, the cancer had still not returned. His doctors told him he had had an uncommonly good outcome, but as his wife put it, 'We lost the old Wilhelm the day he was diagnosed. Who would have imagined depression to be worse than cancer?'

Wilhelm rejected all offers of help. It was obvious to his carers that his deep unhappiness stemmed from the way he held his cancer responsible for everything else that didn't work out in his life. A nurse familiar with him observed, 'He is never angry, he looks just completely defeated and resigned to his imagined fate.'

The shock of a new cancer diagnosis is enough to unsettle a life, let alone an associated termination of a pregnancy, the loss of a business and other complications. A very short-term focus becomes essential for survival. If you are going through cancer treatment, you may be experiencing this situation now. Your goal may be simply getting through breakfast without a hiccup, spending the day without pain or hanging up a load of washing. Even if you know you have bigger things to think about, you may not have the emotional energy to tackle them. Almost everyone I have met resents that small and seemingly inconsequential things like showering, eating and dressing can be time-consuming when you are unwell. 'Don't ask me anything complex,' a weary patient sometimes warned me. 'I spent my brain getting here.' Her attentive husband was her proxy on those occasions.

Anxiety, major and minor depression, low moods and adjustment disorder in cancer are very real dangers. It is thought that between 30 and 40 per cent of patients may experience some symptoms but researchers emphasize that psychological illness is both under-recognized and under-treated. Nevertheless, cancer patients have a significantly higher rate of psychological symptoms than the general population. Whereas women have a higher rate of depression than men in the general population, the rates appear to be more even in cancer patients.

Being periodically worried or upset is normal and, after all, unsurprising after your life has been thrown into turmoil. But when your worries become pervasive and have an impact on your quality of life, your relationships and your work, you need to act.

The first step is to identify what's going on in your mind. Take the chance to reflect on your emotions. Ask those who are close to you to observe some of the changes they have noticed. Don't be afraid of the observations; accepting that emotional upheaval is par for the course, you can start dealing with it. If you can, I'd advise figuring out if there is a particular issue you are troubled by. Does your hand keep going to a lump that you suspect is cancer? Are you worried that you didn't complete all the recommended treatment or that the dose was reduced towards the end? Your oncologist may have altered your treatment plan midway without your understanding why. Or you feel deep down that your doctors are not telling you how things really stand and there's bad news.

A glum-looking patient recently said to me: 'I hate how I look. At one level, I know it's a small price to pay for being alive, but when I look in the mirror, I can't help looking at my scarred chest and my bald head, and feeling despondent. I loved wearing fashionable suits but I just can't be bothered now because I figure everyone knows what's inside.'

Many patients articulate the feelings of despondency about body image that this young man did in the aftermath of intensive treatment. Don't underestimate the upheaval that cancer causes in the way you perceive yourself and how you regard your relationships. It's normal to worry about job security, the capacity to sustain close relationships, and indeed, your survival after cancer treatment.

I am sure there are many others but these are some of the commonest worries that I encounter in patients. Recurrent and deep-seated emotional distress can lead to depression. Some common symptoms of depression include a pervasive feeling of sadness, withdrawal from usually pleasurable activities, sleep difficulties, significant weight shifts, feeling run-down, feeling unmotivated, overwhelmed, hopeless and thinking that life is not worth living. You will note immediately that many cancer patients experience some of these feelings intermittently, which is normal. There is no single checklist to diagnose depression because not every patient experiences every symptom but the key is that if you recognize these or other concerning features on a frequent basis in yourself or your loved one, consider seeking help.

You don't have to be alone in facing your concerns and I would like to emphasize that there are many forms of help available. Some people find relief by sharing their concern with someone they trust and they don't need more formal help. But if you feel awkward doing this because you think they won't understand or that they might worry over you, you can approach your family doctor, oncologist or cancer care nurse to refer you for professional help.

Seeing a psychologist to address set beliefs, fears and anxieties works well for many people without the need for medication. However, for more severe symptoms that are interfering with life, a psychiatrist's advice may help to diagnose and treat an underlying problem such as depression or an adjustment disorder. Prescription medication should be considered an adjunct to psychological help. Counselling and learning ways to change your frame of thinking is a good long-term strategy for better emotional health.

Some patients balk at the thought of adding yet another specialist to their list, both due to cost and inconvenience, but you may not need to see either a psychologist or a psychiatrist permanently. A few sessions may be enough to give you the perspective that your experience is normal and arm you with the right tools. Don't be afraid to acknowledge the need for more intensive help. These days, oncologists can refer patients to psychologists and psychiatrists who deal predominantly with cancer patients and I think there is a benefit to seeing them. Increasingly, hospitals and hospices have a dedicated professional working alongside cancer carers to assist with such cases. The mention of psychiatric help still conveys a stigma to some patients who fear that they will be labelled. In fact, the key reason for seeking psychiatric intervention is to arrest your symptoms, manage them properly, and allow you to resume a normal life.

You may also find a referral to a self-help or support group useful. Some people appreciate hearing from others with a similar experience and find this to be more beneficial than seeking formal help. Trained nurses and doctors periodically attend some groups, providing an opportunity for asking general questions in an informal and supportive environment. It can feel safe to ask seemingly simple questions when you know other people share your view. Again, you don't have to attend sessions indefinitely, only as long as you derive benefit from them.

Keep in mind that a bit like cancer, anxiety and depression affect not only you but those close to you. Many carers describe feeling like helpless bystanders. I hope that if you are not feeling yourself, you too will seriously consider obtaining help. It might change your whole outlook.

Key Points

- Anxiety and depression are common and largely unrecognized in cancer. They are treatable conditions with a great impact on your quality of life.
- Speak up and ask for help if you think you need it – it may change your whole outlook.
- Not everyone needs long-term drug treatment for psychological issues – understanding, acceptance, short-term counselling and other lifestyle measures may suffice. Don't let a dislike of pills or doctors stop you from seeking advice.

23

Does My Oncologist Have Feelings?

Many years ago, Lynn, a dear friend of mine, lost her brother to cancer. George was young, and had aggressive disease with a poor prognosis from the time he was diagnosed. He received chemotherapy, radiotherapy and every other treatment available at the time. But when he died, Lynn was livid with his oncologist.

George's oncologist was not much older than Lynn. When they first met him, he seemed interested in tackling George's disease with all the resources he could muster. Lynn, who had given up work to move in with George, usually brought in a list of things that she had noticed in the preceding weeks, but as George's condition took a turn for the worse, she found the oncologist less and less interested in her accounts.

Two weeks before George died, he acquired pneumonia and went to intensive care where he was intubated and placed on a ventilator. The oncologist did not once speak to Lynn during this time although he dropped in to see George at unannounced hours and would write in his notes. As George lay dying, Lynn was struggling with many questions, many of them to do with the clinical trial he had been on, which in her mind had brought him to this situation. Her elderly mother had early dementia and could become aggressive in her inquiries about George, something Lynn felt helpless to handle. The intensive care doctors talked to her about the day-to-day situation but professed their ignorance of the clinical trial. One suggested that 'it hardly mattered now' and she was wasting her energy.

Lynn made many frustrated interstate calls to me in those weeks. 'I feel as if his oncologist has abandoned us. He was so interested in George earlier but now I feel like he was just a test case. And as soon as he saw George was dying, he just turned away from us. He has moved on to people he can cure.' Lynn made the difficult decision to take George off the ventilator. 'I keep expecting that he has heard George died and he will call me, just to say how sorry he is.' Some weeks later, she announced, 'It has been a month today and I am giving up on receiving any kind of acknowledgement from George's oncologist. I don't care how busy he is, he must have a heart of stone to not see how we all suffered.'

I flinched at the unforgiving description of an oncologist that I had never met. I also knew that any oncologist who had looked after a charismatic patient like George couldn't possibly forget him or not regret his passing away. But I was equally aware that there is a greater than usual expectation that an oncologist will bring to the bedside not just sound technical knowledge but also rich humanistic skills, and, according to Lynn, the latter is where the oncologist had failed.

'I don't care that the surgeon who fished out her appendix was unpleasant because thankfully, we never have to see her again. But I want mum's oncologist to be nice to her. I want him to genuinely care about my mother,' a colleague fretted. I couldn't agree more. In reality, every patient, whether suffering from a burst appendix or advanced cancer, wants to be treated by a doctor who genuinely cares. But it speaks to the depth of the relationship that every patient and carer who has come into contact with an oncologist usually has a strong opinion of him or her.

'I wouldn't be alive without my oncologist', a lady gushed, even as she was admitted to a hospice for terminal care. 'He is a godsend. No matter how late he was running, he would come and visit me in hospital. He always explained why I needed chemo and why it was time to stop. And he always had a smile and a kind word for me, that was the nicest part about seeing him.'

And this from a harried carer: 'I called my oncologist to tell him how sick my husband had suddenly become. I was bowled over when he said, "There is nothing I can do, call an ambulance." I thought he would want to know after five years of seeing him that my husband was dying, that's all. He never saw us again.'

As you read this, you may be one of the many patients or carers who find themselves questioning whether cancer doctors, nurses and other professionals really 'get' it. When you are going through an intense, painful, physically and emotionally rigorous time, it is natural to feel vulnerable.

In these situations, it is also normal for emotions to be polarized. I can't help noticing with my own patients that an almost inadvertent kind gesture on my part becomes magnified and almost mythologized but similarly, a small oversight also becomes exaggerated. It makes me think that where expectations are high, so are disappointments. 'You are an oncologist,' a weary Lynn said once, sighing. 'Just tell me that George's oncologist feels a little bit of my grief because I can't help feeling he is removed from our suffering by a thick wall.'

If you find yourself wondering like poor Lynn about whether your oncologist cares, let me tell you the answer is a resounding yes. I have worked with and met scores of oncologists over the years and I can confidently tell you that they care about you. I can assure you that your circumstances or those of someone like you can keep an oncologist awake some nights, prompt him or her to scour the literature for up-to-date treatments, to send late-night emails to experts, and to corner people at conferences to discuss how best to keep you well.

I remember long before I showed any interest in cancer medicine, an oncologist asking me how I might treat her patient with breast cancer who had progressed after many lines of treatment. Not even able to appreciate the whole problem, I provided some naive answers to which she nodded thoughtfully. Of course she had thought carefully through every option and I now realize that our conversation was her way of reinforcing the sobering conclusion that there was no meaningful chemotherapy remaining for her patient. It was a subtle way of coming to terms with the impending loss of a patient. This doctor, renowned for her bedside manner, would have subsequently returned to her patient, set aside a longer than usual time, and discussed her dilemma openly. She would have dealt with the patient's fears and summoned the best palliative-care resources so that the patient still felt cared for.

However, another oncologist I know might have done things differently in the same situation. He would have discussed the patient's case with others, but then have someone else, like a trainee, deliver the bad news. 'Tell her that there is nothing else we can do but we can put her up for a trial,' he would say. 'But between you and me, I don't think she has got long.'

I suspect that you are immediately unimpressed with the second oncologist's manner. I can just hear the patient's complaint. 'He didn't even have the courtesy to tell me himself, he sent someone junior who didn't have much of an idea.' When I was a trainee, all the trainees knew the oncologists who would sit down and talk with their patients and those who couldn't hide their discomfort at the slightest hint of bad news. I can understand how the latter looks bad to patients but lately, a series of experiences have given me pause to think. A colleague like the second oncologist mentioned above recently lost his young sister to breast cancer. He finds this particular conversation about the end of treatment extremely difficult to have with his breast cancer patients because he becomes visibly upset during the consultation. He finds that his distress exaggerates his patient's distress so temporarily, while he deals with his grief, his way around the problem is by getting someone else to be his proxy. Since I have understood his motivation, his actions don't seem like a dereliction of duty to me. I actually think that in time, his personal experience will make him more attuned to the feelings of his patients but he needs to process his own grief first.

Last year I met a wonderful oncologist, one of the best in her field, who lost her twin brother to a rare cancer. 'His memory is my greatest impetus to spend time in the lab, looking for a cure.' She observed that sometimes her patients must sense her distraction and interpret it as disinterest. But she told me that she is at the risk of losing her marriage because she spends all her time in the laboratory. 'I don't want anyone else to go through my experience. That's why I am always impatient. I hope that one day my patients will forgive this.'

I hope that these stories give you a small insight into the human face of oncologists. I realize that while your oncologist is familiar with minor details of your life, you know almost nothing about his. But remember that cancer is a common condition and it afflicts people indiscriminately. So it is conceivable that your oncologist has either experienced cancer closely in a family member, been worked up for a suspected cancer, or received the diagnosis. I can think of at least three doctors I know who have undergone chemotherapy and are back at work. All these experiences, the reflections of our patients and the expectations of society shape the work of an oncologist.

As I have written elsewhere, I was deeply affected by my grandmother's death from cancer, in particular by the oncologist's lack of discussion around her prognosis. Mind you, he did not refuse to discuss it, it is simply that we never asked and he never told. But the experience left a lasting impact on my family. As a result, when I became an oncologist, I made it a high priority to discuss prognosis and end-of-life care with my patients. I define this as an integral part of my work with the terminally ill. A colleague whose wife had recently emerged from cancer treatment exclaimed, 'All these years of being an oncologist, and I now see cancer through new eyes. I never thought hair loss or broken nails could be so dispiriting to patients but now I see why.'

Another colleague told me that her mother insisted on making every single decision about her chemotherapy although she, the oncologist daughter, could see that some of the decisions were of dubious benefit. 'But when mum died, she said that she was content to have given everything a try. I suspect this memory makes me lenient with some patients who choose to have chemotherapy with minimal benefit. They remind me of my mother and how indignant she would have been if she felt someone had wrested away her autonomy.'

I hope that these anecdotes shine a light on the many motivations that fuel an oncologist. We are, after all, as human as you. While it's rare for oncologists to openly share their doubt, regret or distress with patients, I can tell you that almost every oncologist broods over patients and wonders if things could have been done better or differently. It is part of our job to ponder what could have been. Male or female, seasoned or uninitiated, humble or confident, every oncologist stops to think, and think often, about the patient's plight. I can't tell you the number of times we stop each other in corridors, in elevators, and in the parking lot, to discuss what to do next. Sometimes, it is in search of information, other times it helps to talk. If you are feeling upset about your condition, chances are so is your oncologist. You may be dissatisfied with how he or she expresses it but it might help you believe that deep inside, your oncologist cares.

This is a good place to talk about optimism. Many patients remark that oncologists rarely give effusive praise or demonstrate confident optimism. 'At one year, my oncologist nodded with more worry than I thought was warranted. At two years, she said things were okay. At three years, she still didn't look happy. By five years, I was bouncing with joy and she says, "I think we will bring you back for another five years, you never know."' I can tell you that the same oncologist would count you as one of her success stories and tell everyone about you. It is just that she has also seen many things go wrong and has learnt to be cautious in her public declarations. So don't take the restraint as an insult but rather, a doctor's deliberate instinct to be careful. After all, you want your doctor to do the worrying on your behalf.

In conclusion, I want to assure you again that yes, your oncologist does have feelings, in fact very deep feelings, about the responsibility of a doctor towards some of society's sickest patients. You will not always see these feelings on display for many reasons but in a profession where there is so much choice, those who choose to become oncologists are driven be a desire to eradicate the suffering associated with cancer.

Chances are that in a long journey, you might sometimes question whether your oncologist truly understands and empathizes with your situation. You could ask gently probing questions to ascertain this. If you are deeply and chronically unhappy, you could change oncologists. But I hope that you will simply find consolation in knowing that your oncologist cares about you and that it is a mutually therapeutic journey to help a patient navigate a serious illness with confidence and contentment.

Key Points

- Being a cancer professional is an emotionally intense job – every oncologist has bad days.
- Oncologists think deeply about patient welfare and go to great lengths to find the best management for you.
- Different oncologists express their concern differently; don't mistake lack of communication for disinterest.
- If you are chronically dissatisfied with the way your oncologist engages with you, consider a change.

24

Is My Family at Risk and What Can I Do?

'I know that everyone says I am lucky that my cancer was caught at an early stage and I have an excellent prognosis, but I can't help feeling guilty that I have passed on a genetic weakness to my children.' Sultan was diagnosed with bowel cancer at the age of forty-five, when his twin sons were twelve years old. He had seen his family doctor with anaemia that led to the diagnosis of an early-stage bowel cancer, which was then completely removed. All his close relatives were healthy and lived to old age, so he was baffled by his diagnosis. Sultan had been advised that there was no identifiable hereditary condition responsible for his cancer, a reassurance that both consoled and troubled him in turn.

'I have been running from cancer all my life,' sighed Libby. '"Impressive family history" is the phrase I dread the most. My grandmother, first cousin, mother, sister and niece all have breast cancer, so in a way I wasn't surprised when my turn came. I hate to think that my beautiful sister who just got married is at risk too.' Unlike Sultan, Libby's family was known to carry a genetic mutation associated with a heightened risk of breast and other cancers.

The concerns of Sultan and Libby are very common, but thankfully, most cancers are not inherited and arise as a result of random genetic events. If you have been diagnosed with cancer you are likely to have wondered about the implications for your loved ones. You may also have heard terms such as mutation testing, genetic screening and familial cancer counselling and wonder if they apply to you. Our knowledge in this area is growing and becoming increasingly sophisticated although there is a lot we still don't know and so the advice we can give patients is limited. But I want to spend some time helping you understand cancer genetics and how they might apply to you.

A genetic mutation simply refers to a change in the usual make-up of a gene. A mutation can have beneficial, harmful, neutral or an uncertain effect on your health. Mutations are implicated in not just cancer but a range of other non-cancer conditions, cystic fibrosis, Down's syndrome and colour blindness being some examples.

All cancers result from a mutation but, rather than being inherited from one's parents, most of them are acquired through one's life due to chance, environmental exposure to toxins and other ill-understood factors. Only 5 to 10 per cent of cancers occur due to an inherited genetic defect. Clues to a hereditary cancer syndrome include several affected close relatives, multiple cancers in an individual, when both paired organs (such as breast or kidneys) are involved, an unusual cancer (such as breast cancer in a man), cancers known to be associated with a birth defect and diagnosis at an unusually young age. Sometimes belonging to a certain racial or ethnic group with a known raised risk of cancer may prompt genetic testing.

While their overall number is small, inherited cancers affect diverse organs and it is not just the breast, ovaries and colon that typically receive attention. We currently know of around fifty mutations associated with hereditary cancer syndromes, and genetic testing can reveal whether you possess one of these mutations relevant to your cancer.

If you are a patient with a confirmed cancer diagnosis and your family member is subsequently found to carry the mutation, what does this mean? It is important to understand that carrying a mutation does not mean that a person will develop cancer; rather, it is a marker of increased risk. Some factors that determine whether a mutation leads to cancer include whether the mutation affects one or both copies of the gene, the gender of the carrier, and how completely or strongly a mutation is expressed in an individual. Two people carrying the same mutation do not have the same risk of developing cancer, nor can we say that if they do develop cancer, they will experience it with the same severity.

Obtaining a detailed family history is a vital part of overall cancer care. However, we know that the immediate task of treating the patient at hand consumes most of our early attention. This is reasonable also from a patient's perspective. Genetic testing is time-consuming, so it's likely that both you and your oncologist will turn to a full discussion after the more time-sensitive part of your care has ended. Many oncology services have access to familial cancer centres where geneticists work with oncologists to comprehensively inform patients.

Genetic testing is emerging in India, and is likely to become more prominent with time. Companies are vying to make these tests easy to access, in the privacy of one's home even, simply by collecting a sample of saliva. But Indian experts caution that genetic mutations that apply to Western populations may not be similarly relevant in Indian patients. The whole area of cancer genetics has yet to mature, and better evidence is needed before genetic testing can be widely recommended. This highlights the need for each conversation about genetic risk to be tailored to the individual patient or his healthy relative who chooses to undergo screening.

Genetic testing is typically undertaken with a blood test although the resected tumour specimen can also yield important information. After meticulous processing of the results, the geneticist studies the information. The patient should receive in-depth counselling by a qualified professional before and after the test. Therefore, expect the results to take several weeks to a few months depending on availability and the depth of detail needed.

Genetic testing for a mutation can reveal one of a few answers. A positive result means that a mutation has been identified. If you are a cancer patient, identifying the mutation may inform ongoing treatment, the need for specific risk-reduction measures (such as surgery or medication) or surveillance. If you are a healthy person, it may inform pre-emptive measures including tests and their frequency, preventive surgery or medication and changes to lifestyle such as smoking cessation and weight loss. As explained earlier, a healthy person who tests positive for a mutation will not necessarily develop cancer but a qualified genetic counsellor can advise on the nature of the increased risk.

A negative result means that the specific mutation being tested for was not found. It does not mean that you will never develop cancer or that you don't have another genetic mutation – it just means that the particular test you had did not identify the specific mutation being sought. It is important to understand this point. A negative test is helpful if other close family members affected by cancer are known to carry that mutation, in which case, the absence of a mutation implies that your risk of developing that particular cancer is closer to that of the general population. Sometimes a hereditary cancer is suspected but not proven on genetic testing. A counsellor might explain these issues to you in terms of true and false negative results.

Genetic testing can also yield uncertain results meaning that although a genetic mutation has been identified, we don't know its implications for cancer risk. This may be because no other known person or family has demonstrated the same mutation causing cancer. A result of unknown significance doesn't mean that your geneticist or doctor doesn't know, it indicates the need for more research in the area to arrive at a more definite result.

'When my dad got cancer, I felt this desperate urge to know if I was susceptible to it. I thought that knowledge was power. But when I talked to the counsellors, I realized for the first time that it's not just about getting the result, it's what you plan to do with it and how it affects the rest of your life. I went ahead with it but only after giving it a lot of thought.'

'In retrospect, my son feels he should not have undergone genetic testing. He has found himself in a difficult situation with full disclosure of his genetic history, partly because he never anticipated it.'

'My wife and I have heated arguments about her genetic testing because I don't think the kids need to worry about potential events.'

These are some views I have heard expressed with regard to genetic testing.

By now, I hope you appreciate that, like every single intervention we have talked about in this book, the decision for you or your close relative to undergo genetic testing needs to be thoroughly considered. This means listening closely to the advice from doctors and asking questions. If you are a cancer patient yourself, you should know how genetic testing affects your present and future management. Rather than making each decision as you go along, step back and take a broader view. If the presence of a particular genetic mutation meant a recommendation of preventive surgery or medication and you were firmly against these, should you have the test in the first place? What is the evidence that pre-emptive intervention would reduce your chance of developing cancer? Is the risk reduction large or small and what do the figures really mean for you? As we discussed in Chapter 6, being familiar with absolute and relative risk reduction is helpful.

For some people, knowledge is indeed power but for others it creates anxiety and a sense of helplessness. 'I feel as if I am just waiting for cancer to strike,' sighed a patient. 'Every year that I am free I regard as a bonus, although I know the doctor said nothing of the sort.'

Physicians rely on the person with a mutation to share the details with their close relatives who then have to decide whether they want to be tested. If you are a healthy close relative of a cancer patient, things to consider include what you would do with the information about being a mutation carrier as I have mentioned earlier. What measures are you willing to take to reduce your risk? Be aware that genetic information constitutes health information, which you may be obliged to share with your employer or an insurer for disability or income protection. You may feel a moral imperative to share it with close family members but they may not welcome the information. Consider the impact on you, close relatives and potentially your extended family before testing. It is okay to decline to be tested if after weighing up the advice you feel that the risk is greater than the benefit to you. This is an individual decision guided by your philosophy.

A word here about commercial genetic testing as opposed to genetic testing offered at a medical research or academic centre that is studying cancer. Also called direct-to-consumer tests, commercial tests are advertised in the media and are said to offer customized guidance for decisions involving chemotherapy or medication choices, nutritional needs or dietary supplements. The printouts can look impressive, with pages upon pages of information. There isn't scientific evidence to indicate that these tests provide information beneficial for your clinical care. Since these tests are done without the layer of supervision and expertise that results from consulting an oncologist or genetic counsellor, they may be potentially misleading and confusing.

'I didn't want my patient to pay a few thousand dollars for an unproven genetic test but she insisted on it. It just so happened that the test suggested the chemotherapy I started but it added to the list a range of drugs that I would never use given her other conditions,' an oncologist observed. Therefore, in general, before signing up for unsupervised, inadequately explained and costly tests, remember that there is no substitute for your doctor's clinical judgement and accumulated experience. There are certain approved and quality-controlled genetic tests but their availability is limited in many parts of the world including India. As we have talked about earlier, if you are thinking about having commercial genetic testing, talk to your oncologist whose insight may help shape and inform your decision.

Personalized medicine, or using your unique genetic information to tailor therapy, constitutes the next wave of cancer therapy. Many patients are already deriving benefit from it via new drugs and interventions. Taking the time to understand the implications of genetic testing for you and your family will hopefully open the door to potential benefits without causing unnecessary anxiety or regret.

Key Points

- All cancers result from a mutation but only a very small number of cancer-causing mutations are inherited.
- Certain features such as a strong family history, a very young age of onset and an unusual cancer may trigger suspicion of an inherited cancer.
- Genetic testing and counselling typically takes several weeks to months and it may not be conclusive.
- Think carefully about the implications of testing for you, your job and your family members.
- Be wary of unsupervised genetic tests that are increasingly being marketed directly to consumers. Talk to your oncologist about the value of approved, quality-controlled genetic tests in your case.

25

Handling Unexpected Outcomes

Experience has taught me that no matter how good the planning, communication and execution of cancer care, unexpected things happen. A few things that have gone awry in the lives of some of my patients underscore this lesson.

The first patient was a robust man in his sixties who had recently returned from a holiday in Asia. When he became jaundiced he assumed the suspect was the street food he had indulged in. Eventually, he had some tests that revealed cancer of the colon that heavily involved the liver. He and I had a prolonged discussion about the serious nature of his condition, which would eventually lead to death. However, I reassured him that he was in good shape at the time and should consider having chemotherapy. Never having been ill in his life he couldn't believe his bad luck and expressed a keen desire to receive all possible treatment urgently. I advised him that colon cancer management was a success story in oncology and there were many forms of treatment he could access to keep him well. He and his family were very heartened by the news.

He tolerated several cycles of chemotherapy without problems but then began to suffer fatigue. He wasn't enjoying his garden and stopped playing weekly cards with his friends. He was persistently anaemic and felt faint despite transfusions. He then developed other side effects that wore him down. It was clear that a break from treatment was warranted. I told him that recent scans showed the disease was stable and this was a good time to have a break. However, he had read on a blog that he should receive at least six months of chemotherapy before taking a break and consequently felt uncomfortable accepting my advice. 'It's not that I doubt you,' he offered, 'but I've made it to five months and want to push on.' With the help of his equally tenacious wife he persuaded me to prescribe just one more cycle of chemotherapy to help him achieve his goal. I faced a dilemma but eventually felt satisfied that he understood my concerns. In cases like this it's difficult to offer a flat refusal, because they are 'borderline' calls that rely strongly on the judgement of both doctor and patient. I did, however, reduce the dose of chemo and insisted that I would have to assess him carefully before prescribing any more treatment. Having won his current fight he dismissed my concern and agreed to return soon.

On the day of chemotherapy he looked tired but told the nurse that he was always so. His blood tests were just at the level to enable him to proceed with chemotherapy. However, only days after treatment he became severely unwell. By the time he presented himself to the hospital he was off-balance with a very low blood pressure. He was diagnosed with severe pneumonia. He was admitted to the high-dependency unit, where no amount of aggressive antibiotics and blood pressure support could save his life.

His wife revealed tearfully that although he had pushed himself to receive treatment he had never contemplated that one more cycle of chemotherapy could be fatal. 'He told me that he expected to feel the usual nausea, lack of appetite and fatigue but then it would be over and he would have made it to the six-month mark. Then he had every intention of having a break on a long-planned cruise.' Crestfallen, she reflected, 'I wish you had told him he could die.'

'I didn't expect him to die, either,' I explained gently. 'He was used to the chemotherapy and insisted on having more, and I reduced the dose out of caution. I feel bad that I didn't insist on his stopping, but I found it hard to dampen his enthusiasm.'

In his wake, the patient left a mountain of unpaid bills and incomplete paperwork, which took his wife and two children the best part of a year to tackle. They found the task stressful and painful and at times spoke of feeling resentful that he had abandoned them prematurely.

Pneumonia is a serious illness that doesn't require the aid of toxic chemotherapy to cause harm, or even death. But I couldn't help feeling a sense of a missed opportunity to rehabilitate his quality of life for a while longer rather than send him to his death. Ironically, the patient and I had discussed death and dying on two occasions. But both times, we had spoken of the 'normal' process of dying. He expected that one day I would reveal his chemotherapy to be no longer working. He would experience more fatigue and pain and would become more housebound. Slowly his consciousness would fade and he would be transferred to a hospice for end-of-life care, because he didn't want to die in the house his wife would continue to inhabit. He assumed that there would be an interval of days to weeks as this process unfolded, and he would continue to attend to his final wishes during this time. Alas, he didn't ever bank on a relatively sudden death due to acute complications.

The second patient was a young woman with gastric cancer, which was diagnosed at a stage when the surgeon deemed it curable. A cure necessitated chemotherapy followed by surgery to remove part of her stomach. The original plan was for the patient to receive some cycles of chemotherapy followed by an operation, as is the standard protocol. A non-smoker and teetotaller with four young children, she was stunned at the news of her cancer but relieved that the surgeon sounded confident about a cure. She'd been told to expect a number of side effects from the traditional combination of drugs, and in preparation for being temporarily unwell she recruited some of her friends to help.

Nothing prepared her for the devastating outcome following the very first dose of chemotherapy. The cancer began to bleed profusely and she was admitted to hospital in a state of shock. She went to the operation theatre at midnight and emerged at dawn with her entire stomach having been removed to stem a catastrophic bleed. She spent weeks in the intensive care unit and lost half her body weight. On discharge, she fatigued very easily and had to be helped with even small tasks. With her stomach removed, she had trouble eating large amounts, so she had supplemental tube feeding for a year. Her husband left work to look after her and her youngest children relied on the older two to see them through many needs.

A patient like her would have benefited from chemotherapy to remove any remaining trace of tumour but she was in no shape to have it. In response to her doctors' worry, she not only had to make peace with her desperately wasted condition but also the fact that the disease would surely return with a vengeance.

Incredibly, many years have passed since those grim pronouncements and the patient has not only survived, she looks better with every passing year. She is eating and drinking normally although she can only handle small quantities at a time, and participates in a full life with her children. Her husband is still a diligent and devoted carer but she is no longer dependent on him. Whenever I see them, the couple express wonder at her survival. Her surgeon and I are also both amazed at her well-being – neither of us was brave enough to predict this. The patient never expected that she could bleed to near-death following a single cycle of chemotherapy because no one else expected it. Yet when it happened, it made sense as one of many adverse effects that could have occurred.

The fact is that so many things can go wrong during cancer treatment that it is impossible to predict all of them. The list would be interminable for the doctor and so endlessly worrying for the patient that it would achieve nothing.

The fate of these two patients is no doubt sobering, but the lesson that I would take away from their account is that it's important to expect the unexpected when having cancer treatment. As a cancer patient you understand that you have a serious illness. Increasingly improved diagnostics allow doctors a much better insight into cancer, and hence, a greater ability to predict things that could go wrong. For example, mapping the location of bony spread of cancer can help predict an area of impending fracture, which can be repaired in advance, thus avoiding pain and complications. Precisely locating a cancer with new technology means the surgeon has a better sense of the operative technique required. Better and more specific drugs means that we are able to target cancer more accurately than ever before. Newer forms of radiation therapy allow us to treat a tumour without inflicting too much surrounding damage. Thanks to modern technology, we also know far more about adverse effects and how to prevent, manage and treat them. This also means that your oncologist has hopefully spoken to you about some potential obstacles that could occur in your care. For example, knowing that a patient of mine had a particular type and location of lung cancer, I advised him that there was a strong possibility that the cancer could bleed. He had a strong view against resuscitation in this instance, which was useful to know and record.

Nonetheless, the truth is that unexpected outcomes will occur despite the best preparation. It is not anyone's fault but related to the vagaries of the human body.

My advice to all patients is to expect the best, but understand that things can go wrong suddenly. It's hard to always be in a complete state of readiness for something to go wrong, but small and important ways of preparing include taking care of your advance-care directive, and your will, when you're feeling well and can think clearly. An advance-care directive is a document that states your wishes for medical care if you are unable to articulate those decisions at any time. We will spend more time discussing this in Chapter 30.

Make sure your strongest wishes, whether to do with your business, house or funeral, are known to those close to you. If you can't run your business any more, is there someone who can step in? Where are the most important papers associated with the business that a new person might need immediately? If there are outstanding finances relating to your house or other properties, does someone understand this and know where to turn next? Consider documenting important passwords or assigning a trusted person as your power of attorney to act on your behalf.

I recall a woman who cycled between deep sorrow and great bitterness at the loss of her husband. Although he had been unwell for four years, he had steadfastly maintained control of his vast business interests. 'He always promised to let me know where everything was and a priority list of what to do but he never got to it because he didn't want to think about dying. And when he died, our children and I felt drowned by the paperwork. He didn't leave us in debt or anything bad, and he had appointed a manager, but the manager assumed I had some knowledge. The children and I felt very angry with my husband for inflicting this further pain upon us.'

If you have particular instructions for your funeral, make sure someone knows them. I once looked after a patient who meticulously documented a guest list and wrote a lovely letter of reflection and gratitude to be opened at the funeral by his friend. His wife felt consoled by his strong presence at the gathering. Remember that routine things such as your banking, personal, or business dealings, may be completely unfamiliar to your spouse or children. Begin by listing important details on paper. A good tip a former patient gave me is that he would stand in every room and think about the things he would need to tell somebody about to lease his house. He wrote down where the meters and lines were, security passwords, how to operate the pool, which neighbours were reliable, and other things that were second nature to him after thirty years.

Be aware of your condition and learn to listen to your body. If you're not feeling well, don't deny it to yourself. If you have a sense that things are not working out, talk it over with an expert. Many cancer patients are naturally anxious, but don't dismiss your anxiety, rather work on it. Even in an age of saturation with information, your gut instinct is crucial – cultivate it.

If you are a carer, you can help the patient by gently introducing some admittedly difficult concepts into your conversation. Many patients secretly fear the worst but don't mention it for fear of upsetting their loved ones. You might want to signal to the patient that you are prepared to listen to serious reflections and decisions – this may be the green light the patient needs. Remember that a carer's worries are eased in the long term if he is not always guessing the patient's intentions.

Unexpected outcomes such as disease recurrence despite the expectation of being cured, difficult-to-control symptoms, serious disability or untimely death are unfortunately a part of the journey of life. They don't happen only to cancer patients but to all kinds of people. A perfectly normal pregnancy suddenly goes wrong, a mildly overweight driver has a devastating stroke in the middle of the highway, and an elite athlete drops dead of a cardiac arrest. You, your oncologist and other carers can manage risk, but you can never eliminate it. This is why it's important to keep adjusting expectations in tune with your circumstances and accept that, despite the vast reach of modern medicine, unexpected things will happen. It pays to put your mind in advance to how best you or your loved one might handle them.

Key Points

- Despite careful preparation unexpected outcomes happen in cancer as they do in life. They are nobody's fault.
- Unexpected and disappointing outcomes in cancer may include no response to treatment, rapidly advancing disease, severe bleeding, infection or an early death. These are difficult considerations for everyone, which makes having an advance-care directive really important.
- Patients who are prepared to confront difficult questions about their life and discuss them with their family render them a valuable service because they are informed about the patient's choices.

26

How Long Do I Have?

'The first time I heard the word *cancer* all I had going through my mind was "How long?" I didn't hear a single thing the doctor said.'

For many people, particularly those diagnosed with incurable cancer, this is the question that dominates the course of their journey. Yet we know from anecdotes as well as formal research that conveying prognosis to cancer patients is an area that too often suffers from inadequate doctor–patient communication.

'If she doesn't have long, some days I really want to know,' a carer put it succinctly, 'and on other days, I want to run away from the knowledge. But mostly, I think she needs to know – it's only fair.'

I imagine that if you or someone close to you has cancer these comments will resonate. Although cancer prognosis varies greatly depending upon the affected organ, the stage of the disease and many other factors (such as other serious illnesses you have), it is quite common to equate cancer with dying. This fear figures heavily on patient's minds. So in some ways it is quite remarkable that more patients don't ask about prognosis more often. It is even more remarkable how many patients don't ask at all, even when they suspect they don't have long to live and privately long to know. Regrettably, the matter is not discussed as often as it should because it is difficult and sensitive for both doctor and patient.

As someone who has been on the receiving end of secrecy surrounding cancer prognosis, I recall that my family made many of the decisions about my ill grandmother in a vacuum of knowledge. This was at the age of ten, well before my own medical studies, when I had as little understanding of the process as anyone else in the family. Her oncologist simply shook his head outside her room, telling us there was no hope. Her usually healthy complexion was stained by severe jaundice and her renowned stamina had seemingly dissipated overnight. A matriarch who liked nothing better than to chat, her capacity for words grew heartbreakingly small as all she could do was rouse herself from sleep time to time, smile weakly and acknowledge our presence with a flicker of her hand. A perpetual drip hung from her dainty arm. Sometimes we surmised there was chemotherapy in it and other times saline. Her food trays were sent back untouched as she expressed a general distaste for food.

When her advanced cancer was diagnosed, my grandmother found herself in a hospital that had some of the best cancer services of the time. But she was far away from home in a foreign city where, despite the presence of her children, she never felt at home. She was caged by the four walls of her small hospital room, not permitted to visit home, as was the custom of the day. The sad thing is that she wasn't really receiving any worthwhile treatment in the hospital because the oncologist had said that her cancer was too advanced for cure, and anyway, no good chemotherapy existed for it. But because he didn't suggest it and my family was too overwhelmed with the day-to-day logistics of her care, nobody ever broached the issue of going home to die, which might just have brought with it some form of a discussion about prognosis.

My grandmother was an extremely devout woman whose daily life revolved around praying for her family's welfare. Although I was too young to have these exchanges with her, from all that I remember of her and the snippets of conversation that the adults had, I know that she would have preferred nothing better than to go home to die in peace. Informed of the gravity of her situation, I suspect she would have been initially upset, because here was a woman who had throughout her life eaten healthily and exercised regularly and still had things to take care of. She knew how to make peace with the vicissitudes of life. And if all else failed, she had a robust faith that would have helped her accept her fate as God's will. I imagine that she would have liked to have spent her last few weeks praying to her God and sorting out the mementos that she wanted her many children and grandchildren to remember her by. As it happened, she died in her hospital room, with none of these wishes fulfilled.

Thirty years on we console ourselves that she realized she was sick and that the hospital was the best place to be. But regarding the situation through the eyes of the oncologist I have become, I see that there was nothing that the hospital did for her that could not have been reproduced at home. She didn't have complex pain management or other medical or mobility issues that can legitimately delay or prevent some people from going home. She had a full-time carer or family member sitting with her day and night, which would have been much easier to do at home. Towards the end of her life, she sunk into a coma before slipping away peacefully. She was cremated in a foreign city.

While of course no one can say for sure – and my grandmother was certainly the most obliging and selfless person I ever knew and might well have gone along with what was easiest – I cannot help thinking that if posed the question, 'Where and how would you like to spend your last days?', she would have said, 'At home.'

When we talk as a family about her death, it is still with a hint of regret. We mourn her early death, of course, but also that things happened under the cover of darkness. She was never told her diagnosis, although I bet she knew. Everyone pretended to be upbeat as if nothing was wrong and the hospitalization was temporary. There was no time for any meaningful conversation – the kind you have with a pain in your insides, knowing it's your last. When she died, it was almost as if we were asking for the first time, 'What just happened?' We consoled ourselves that we did the best we could. And perhaps we did, given the times.

Today, thirty years later, as an oncologist, I still see variations of the same theme. Of all the things that patients feel dissatisfied with, communication around the end of life is writ large. So many things have improved in cancer medicine but improvement in communication has been regrettably slow to keep pace.

In studies, the majority of cancer patients tell us that they want to know how long they have to live because it helps them define their goals of care and order their priorities. They tell us that rather than diminishing or stealing hope, knowing their prognosis helps them deal with their worst fears and allows them to live life meaningfully. When they are reassured of their doctor's support they actually describe feeling hopeful about their future, not more depressed as we customarily imagine. When those who advocate not telling cancer patients about prognosis are asked what their own preference would be in the circumstances, they say they would like to be told the truth.

Since this is such an important aspect of your cancer care, I would like to talk to you about how you might discuss your prognosis with your oncologist.

When cancer is in remission, the discussion is easier. The oncologist will be quite happy to tell you, for example, that people like you have a 95 per cent likelihood of being cured although vigilance needs to be maintained. A body of literature about cure rates, chance of relapse and long-term issues for survivors can enlighten this conversation. To be honest, the majority of people are so relieved to hear the good news that they seldom quibble about 'the missing 5 per cent that I could cry over' as my patient with a curable cancer pointed out with a smile.

The discussion about prognosis is more unpalatable, yet more urgent, for those with advanced cancer. Some oncologists consider it an important pillar of their role to routinely broach prognosis with their patients when the time is right. Typical opportunities might arise when multiple lines of chemotherapy have failed, the patient shows clinical deterioration, or when a patient expresses a wish to know what the future holds. The oncologist will set aside a time, invite other family members to attend a meeting, and deal with questions and doubts with patience, empathy, and understanding. This kind of interaction frequently leaves doctors and patients feeling better.

However, as many patients and families continue to report, for far too many patients, the discussion about prognosis is unplanned and unstructured. For some it is completely incidental. 'I told my doctor that I couldn't wait to finish chemotherapy to go fishing, and he said, "Theoretically, you could be on this forever," which triggered a conversation I wasn't expecting to have, although I am glad I did.'

Sometime ago a patient signalled her ambivalence regarding further chemotherapy because of the side effects she was experiencing. I told her that indeed, the chemotherapy was not doing her any favours. Our conversation then drifted towards maximizing quality of life and in a roundabout way, we reached a discussion about prognosis.

Many patients land in an emergency room one night, where an

unfamiliar, busy and admittedly, often unwilling, doctor must chat to them about their wishes for resuscitation, leading to a discussion about the usually guarded prognosis. No one thinks that this is a proper way to find out such important information; it's something every oncologist should strive for a patient to avoid.

As you can see, some patients become aware of their prognosis in appropriate circumstances and others not. For far too many people, the whole issue remains unspoken because it's too confrontational.

I know of some patients who are determined in their desire to live every day of life well without being interested in prognosis – they are a small subset, whose wishes should obviously be respected. But many more people are similarly interested in living a good life accompanied by an idea of how long they have to do it. They express a wish to tie up various aspects of modern-day life – from financial planning to the finishing touches to a tree house, from arranging a family gathering to noting down a list of banking passwords. This surely sounds reasonable too.

Assuming that you are interested in knowing roughly how long you have to live, what happens when you ask your oncologist? Some oncologists provide an estimate and talk their patients through what this means. But regrettably, all too often, patients describe not receiving a direct answer. One weary patient put it thus: 'She kept telling me she didn't know and that cancer is one of those conditions where no one knows.' Another man said, 'I said I didn't want an exact week or anything but some broad idea, but the doctor looked uncomfortable and said that was not something I needed to think about right now.' Many patients report being implicitly discouraged from considering prognosis. 'My doctor says, "Now, let's be positive", but there is nothing pessimistic about asking to know the details, I just want a sense of control.'

One husband described his repeated attempt to obtain information on behalf of his wife. 'Towards the end, it was clear that switching chemotherapy drugs was not the answer. The oncologist needed to tell my wife that things were heading in the wrong direction, and I hinted at this by saying things like, "What is the short-term outlook?" or "Do you think more treatment will really change things?", but the doctor always took the literal meaning of my questions. I found it impossible to steer the conversation. As I feared, she died on chemo and we never had a chance to stop and take stock of our lives.'

Why is it difficult for an oncologist to discuss prognosis? Let me tell you the two reasons that I personally struggle with, which I think I share with the wider medical profession.

When someone asks me how long he has, my first thought is 'I don't know'. Well, this is a little bit true and a little bit untrue. From the benefit of experience I have a reasonable idea about how a patient will fare. My estimation is supported by knowing the tumour details but mostly by watching patient factors, such as response to treatment, setbacks suffered and ongoing symptoms as well as how much stress other organs are under. This kind of database of experience built over time is very helpful in forming a big picture. In a way, this is pattern recognition, a common way doctors learn, and the more experience you accumulate the more patterns you see.

Doctors who don't agree with this approach contend that although there is more information than ever about predicting prognosis, our ability to take this data from a big population and apply it to an individual patient is not good. This is because an individual is just that – everyone varies in the way their body works and their cancer behaves. You may have come across other people with the same cancer – these days, the Internet allows patients to connect through news articles, advertisements, blogs and chat rooms, not to mention concerned family and friends. My patients sometimes tell me about someone just like them and ask why they were given a different prognosis. I explain that in subtle ways every cancer patient is unique and they shouldn't assume otherwise. However, while it's true that no two patients behave in *exactly* the same way, I don't believe that it should be an excuse for doctors to avoid providing the best possible customized advice on your prognosis.

I don't know anyone who finds discussing a bad prognosis easy. I often begin the conversation by advising patients that while I can't be absolutely sure I will use the best of my knowledge about their case to estimate their prognosis, which is different from taking an entirely random guess. One way of estimating prognosis is to divide it broadly into 'months to years', 'weeks to months' and 'days to weeks'. I find this breakdown a useful way of communicating grave news, with the caveat that things can and do change suddenly. For example, someone who looks okay can deteriorate rapidly at home and I may not have the chance to see him again to revise my prognosis. Palliative-care nurses are valuable in detecting changes in a patient's condition and advising the family. Just as people can deteriorate unexpectedly, a medication can surprise us by stabilizing symptoms, in which case also the prognosis might alter.

As an oncologist it's important to recognize uncertainty but convey it effectively to patients to help them plan ahead. I must admit that it is only with growing older that I've become comfortable with uncertainty myself, which has in turn made it easier to share what I know as well as what I don't know about a disease. I'm always pleasantly surprised by how well patients respond to an honest admission of uncertainty on my part, especially when it is accompanied by a reassurance that I will continue to finesse my advice. It seems a safe bet that if your doctor is an open communicator, you'll be more understanding of his or her uncertainty.

A very important part of understanding your prognosis is to accept the uncertainty inherent in it. No amount of literature or second opinions will remove every ounce of uncertainty and you should avoid dogmatic pronunciations. A comatose patient may be expected to live for only a few days but I have seen patients die within hours as well as survive nearly a fortnight. Age, type of disease, supplemental feeding, other illnesses, intravenous hydration and sedation, and other considerations are important but they have not always helped doctors distinguish between the two outcomes.

I should mention that prognosis is not to be equated with death. Many people with a cure or remission rightly worry about their prognosis too. In another example, imagine someone quoting the latest research that shows five out of ten patients with your condition would be expected to have a recurrence within one year. This also means five patients will be safe from a recurrence. 'Well, which one of those ten am I?' is a reasonable question that a frustrated patient might ask. There is no test that can reliably provide an answer but an oncologist can explain how he might monitor you for signs of recurrence. I feel that the majority of patients accept this explanation; what they like less is when their doctor just says, 'I have no idea.' Patients justifiably expect their oncologist to be more informed than that.

Uncertainty is emotionally difficult but it is no one's fault, and indeed, it is part of many other aspects of life. You don't know if your company is going to retrench you next year. And you don't know whether your daughter's marriage will withstand the stresses she is under. You don't know whether the fierce storm will damage your house or your neighbour's. You do your best to insulate yourself against mishaps but if you modify your expectations and don't expect a precise answer to every question, you can save yourself and your loved ones a lot of anxiety and discontent.

One of my patients who had long believed that she was dying was thrilled to hear of her remission and the fact that her oncologist declared her 'as safe as he had seen the best of patients'. One man married his long-term girlfriend earlier when he was told he may have less time on his hands. So I hope you see that where there is uncertainty doctors and patients can work together to deal with it.

If the first reason doctors don't discuss prognosis is because of uncertainty, the other important reason may be easier to sympathize with – no one likes giving bad news, especially not doctors who are charged with keeping hope alive. As one doctor put it, 'I just hate telling patients there is nothing more.' Your oncologist doesn't like telling you that things are not as bright as you believe, or worse, that you don't have long to live. Obligatory as the task sounds to patients, it is unpleasant and no doctor wants to be seen as the one who crushes hope. Medical training centres that treate illness and cure people have come a long way in doing just that. To admit that there is nothing else one can do for a patient flies in the face of all that doctors are taught.

Although there is growing recognition within the medical profession that we need to equip doctors better to handle sensitive conversations, most doctors still learn to have these conversations by trial and error. Given the frequent sense of disappointment and personal failure during this time, and a doctor's own anxiety about handling uncertainty, it is understandable why many doctors prefer to sidestep this issue. I hope that this partly explains why many doctors look and feel awkward when discussing bad news. But we now know that we can provide doctors with tools and checklists and hone their skills in communicating good and bad news.

I share the difficulties of prognosis with you not to dissuade you from asking about it, but to give you a better understanding of what goes on in your oncologist's mind when you do. Let's now return to how you can help yourself or your loved one.

Think about why you wish to know your prognosis and how you might utilize the information. Knowing that your prognosis is good might give you the boost you need to get to the finish line. On the other hand, your oncologist saying that the prognosis is not greatly altered by chemotherapy may be the information you need to stop treatment and have a quiet holiday. Your child might use that information to bring her wedding forward or you may decide that the time to spend some of your savings is now. Writing down what's important to you can help. You might actually just want to know that the oncologist can keep you comfortable and pain-free, without needing a time frame. Or, for reasons mentioned above, you might prefer a time frame, understanding it can only be an estimate.

Ask your doctor openly. Consider reassuring him or her that you are only asking for a reasonable estimate rather than a figure he or she will be forever held to. If there is an event or a person that features strongly in your reasons, share it with your doctor. Even doctors who have previously avoided discussing prognosis may be moved to consider whether your husband will make it to your son's graduation in three months or whether you will attend your grandchild's first birthday in two weeks. Remember that your doctor genuinely wants to ease your burden – help him or her do this.

You are entitled to seek a second opinion if you cannot get any answer about prognosis. There's a difference between seeking a more favourable answer and not having one at all. Remember that where there is uncertainty, doctors can be variously circumspect. One doctor might think that a 50 per cent chance of survival in the next year is very good. Another will regard it in terms of half his patients dying that year and consider it a bad outcome. We know that the closer your relationship with your doctor the more he or she might overestimate your prognosis, conceivably because it is hard to let go. Think how testing it might be for your doctor to have treated you and grow attached to you, and then be entirely objective about your prognosis – after all, it is human for us all to hope that things were different. However, if you're getting nowhere, it's reasonable to find another source of information, which might be another oncologist, your family doctor or yet another doctor closely involved in your care.

When I think back above all my patients who have asked about their prognosis and how they have reacted, I can say that those who had allowed themselves to contemplate their mortality seemed more accepting of bad news. They had been coming to terms with the matter for some time and my news served to confirm their thoughts. Many have said they felt relieved that I had confirmed their suspicion and reassured that there was good supportive care available to help them through the future.

The patient who reacted most vehemently to a dismal prognosis did so because she believed that no one had told her that she had advanced cancer that was incurable. By the time I had entered the picture of her treatment and told her truthfully that I felt she had weeks to live, she reacted with fury. Her oncologist said that the patient had never been ready to discuss prognosis, so he had hesitated to mention it.

My advice is that you know by now that cancer is a bruising encounter. There are exciting advances occurring and more people are surviving the diagnosis. Your journey depends partly on emotional resilience. Try to prepare yourself for serious news but don't let it dictate your whole life. If you are cured or are in a remission, do your best to live normally. If you are more ill, understand that there is genuine uncertainty in predicting prognosis and don't take it personally when your oncologist doesn't seem eager to discuss it. However, don't assume that your oncologist can't or won't talk about it. The best thing to do is to ask. Tell your oncologist why it is important to you and what you would do with the information. Reassure him or her that you understand the answer might change. And by all means, obtain a second opinion if it helps you.

I empathize that this advice is easy for me to dispense and harder for you to implement. But thinking through some of the issues I have identified might just help you live well through uncertain times.

Key Points

- You have a right to know as much as possible about your prognosis whether you are cured or have advanced illness, because it helps you determine goals in life.
- A prognosis may not be entirely accurate but a frank and sensitive discussion with your oncologist can go a long way towards helping you decide on vital aspects of your future.
- Don't be afraid to ask directly about your prognosis and mention why it's important for you to know. Families try to protect patients from bad news – tell them too why it matters to you.
- You can determine when and how much you want to be told. You can determine whom you want to be present with you for difficult conversations.

27

What Is Palliative Care?

'No,' he says, shaking his head vigorously. 'These things are not for me.'

'But ...' I start.

'Palliative care is for dying people,' he declares. 'I have no plans to die.' His wife looks on helplessly. His daughter sighs.

Terry has been a robust farmer whose favourite description of himself is 'as tough as a bull'. He has kept a sprawling farm properly afloat in difficult conditions, through severe drought, diminishing profits and the departure of many disheartened farmhands who have left for the city in search of better opportunity. Several times over the last few years, his family has encouraged him to sell the property, but he won't hear of it and continues to play a very active role in managing it.

The diagnosis of prostate cancer three years ago tempered Terry's zest for a few months but no sooner had his pain controlled and a treatment regimen decided than he went back to doing what he loved best. Until recently he has kept reasonably well and attributed his health to keeping busy on the farm. But the last few months have seen him deteriorate. The pain keeps coming back in different places and his appetite is failing. His clothes are becoming loose, and despite his deep interest in his farm, he finds himself less and less able to perform any sustained activity. 'You can't tell the cattle to wait until your afternoon nap,' he grumbles.

Six weeks ago, his eldest daughter convinced him to move from the country into her house for a short time. He didn't like the idea but saw the wisdom of it when he realized he was requiring a specialist appointment every week to monitor his symptoms. Now he needs radiotherapy to his painful spine and it's much more convenient for him to stay with his daughter than to travel back and forth to hospital. In a private phone call, his wife advised me that she no longer feels comfortable staying at the farm with her husband, due to the lack of social and medical supports.

'When Terry gets painful spasms, I panic,' she said. 'It's only my daughter's calm voice on the phone that gets me through.'

Terry's daughter has a large house with two adult children who are very helpful, and the whole family feels that Terry and his wife would best be served remaining there. 'The sticking point is Dad, doctor,' the daughter told me. 'We can all see it, but he just doesn't want to face the reality. Maybe you can persuade him.'

At our consultation, I press the case with him. 'Terry, I know you're not dying, but palliative care can help you live better.'

'I'm fine' he says, waving his hand dismissively.

'No you're not, Dad,' his daughter says, sighing. 'Three days this week, you have had such bad pain that we've had to help you back to bed. It would be so nice to know that we can call on someone for help if it happens again.'

'The radiation will fix the pain. I promise you it won't happen again,' he says, with what he intends as a reassuring wink.

'Terry, tell me what you understand about palliative care,' I ask him.

'Look, love, I know you're my doctor, but I tell you palliative care is for people whom you give up on. I want you to keep fighting my cancer. I have my farm to get back to.'

'An introduction to palliative care won't mean the end of my care, but an extension of this care into your home, Terry. The nurses can monitor your pain, for example, and detect emergencies before they occur. They can also alert me of their concerns before you get worse.'

'They'll just give me morphine,' Terry says. 'And I'm not ready for that yet.'

'I know you like details. Can I give you a brochure about community palliative care? You can read it and get back to me.'

'And if I still say no?'

'Terry, don't be so rude!' his wife exclaims. 'The doctor is only trying to help.'

'If you don't think it's for you, I won't impose it on you, Terry. I promise.'

Reassured, he goes home. Later, his daughter calls me to apologize for her father's reluctance to accept help. 'His own father lived to ninety-eight and Dad can't believe he's only seventy-six and ill. He often says that his dad died when he accepted the doctor's offer to have a nurse come into his house to dress an ulcer. He says that Grandpa lost the will to live when he saw that he was dependent on nurses.'

I reassure Terry's daughter that it often takes patients time to reconcile to a change in their condition and accept palliative-care support. Indeed, Terry declines to participate in the conversation for another three weeks, during which time I continue to manage his symptoms in the office and via phone calls.

Then one day he suddenly offers, 'You know, doc, I've been thinking about palliative care and I feel I might as well let them in.'

I ask him gently what changed his mind.

'Time,' he says. 'I just needed my own time to figure out that I am getting worse and having me at home is hard enough for my family without putting an extra weight on them to be on alert all the time. I also talked to my doctor, who convinced me that palliative care is a good thing. I guess I was just being a stubborn old bull, doc.'

The palliative-care nurses make a start, escalating their visits from once weekly to twice a week as Terry's needs increase. They introduce him to a volunteer who helps him record a legacy, like a written or taped interview for his grandchildren, something he enjoys making. Although he continues to deteriorate physically, they manage to keep him comfortable until the end. In his last few days, Terry becomes breathless and expresses a wish to not die at home because he doesn't want his grandchildren to be affected by the experience. The palliative-care nurses arrange for Terry to be transferred to a hospice where he dies peacefully.

Later, Terry's family expresses their gratitude and relief that he accepted the services of palliative care. 'We were never going to tell him, but it was incredibly stressful being his family as well as medical support when he had severe pain. We were terrified of getting something wrong and the palliative-care backup preserved our sanity.'

If you have cancer and are within reach of a palliative-care service, count yourself fortunate. This team of doctors, nurses, social workers, counsellors, volunteers and others is a relatively recent concept in medical care that is now taking the world stage. Why? Because cancer professionals are recognizing that if we truly want to provide comprehensive care to cancer patients, we have to go beyond chemotherapy. We must manage the significant symptoms of cancer, physical and psychological, *and* maximize quality of life in a holistic way. This means helping people stay in their home or comfortable environment as much as possible and respecting their wishes about the direction of their care.

Palliative-care health professionals manage symptoms such as pain, anxiety and nausea, but often also have a better overview of your capacity to manage at home, the level of support you need, and what changes will improve quality of life. It is not that your oncologist cannot manage all these things, but that one person is usually not enough. Depending on how well you are and where you live, palliative care can be delivered in your home or a dedicated centre like a hospice. A hospice has a limited number of beds and is reserved for people with the most critical needs. For many patients, home-based care is the practical, appropriate and favoured option.

If you have advanced cancer, increasingly your oncologist, family doctor or other professional, such as a nurse or social worker, will suggest a palliative-care referral. The pattern of referral varies. Some doctors have a policy of referring all newly diagnosed cases of advanced cancer, anticipating that the patient will eventually need some form of help. Other doctors reserve palliative-care input until later, perhaps when there is a specific symptom they think needs management. There is no right or wrong way as long as you get the help in a timely fashion, remembering that there can be a delay between referral and consultation. If you believe you could do with palliative-care input, don't hesitate to ask.

Palliative-care nurses are highly trained. Depending on the format used in your region, a nurse will conduct an initial visit to your house to discuss your illness, troublesome symptoms and how best the team can help you stay well. It's important to be open and honest with the nurse to get the most appropriate help. For example, if you are having trouble walking, don't hide it from the nurse, who may suggest a frame or ways in which you can reduce the need to walk. Similarly, freely discussing pain or loss of weight is important, without fearing that the nurse is there to take away your independence by recommending hospitalization. Remember that palliative-care workers respect your wish to be at home and will work hard with you to make that possible.

After the initial visit, your ongoing need determines the frequency of nurse visits. Some services have a phone outreach programme so that you can call for advice. Their ability to come out to you at unscheduled times depends on the specific programme, but sometimes simply having someone trusted offering advice is enough. The nurse might also suggest or arrange other services, and will liaise with your doctor, psychologist and so on.

A small number of patients introduced to palliative care are admitted directly to a hospice, which is sometimes located on hospital grounds but has a different model of care. Like home palliative care, a hospice concentrates on preserving quality of life rather than tests and interventions. Being admitted to a palliative-care service doesn't mean that you can never have a test again but in general, the emphasis will be on avoiding them because tests can cause pain and anxiety and not alter your overall condition. You might be admitted to a hospice if you are too weak or unwell to go home from hospital, or if your pain relief or other symptom management requires round-the-clock supervision. Again, you will only go to a hospice with your consent and if you don't enter a hospice, you can still receive appropriate care from the palliative-care team.

Contrary to common belief, not everyone goes to a hospice to die and not everyone in a hospice has cancer. Many patients enter a hospice for a period of respite or symptom management. If pain is disrupting your life, a stint in a hospice may stabilize it and allow you to get home again. Some people are admitted to a hospice because their carer needs a rest. You should go to a hospice with an open mind – if you improve you can return home, but if you deteriorate, there is a backup. Unfortunately, there are not nearly enough palliative-care beds in hospitals or hospices to meet the needs of all the patients who need them but the palliative-care services that I have worked with have been very experienced at prioritizing the needs of patients.

Having seen many patients benefit, I am an enthusiastic supporter of palliative-care supports. Although I feel comfortable managing a range of symptoms I always feel at ease when I know my patients have another, home-based support. I find the phone calls and updates from palliative care useful and their visits often prevent unnecessary emergency room dashes and hospitalization.

Unlike what you may have heard, palliative care does not expedite death. It aims to make the final phase of life more comfortable and pain-free, and eases the burden on your loved ones. Recent research indicates that early introduction to palliative care might even help some patients live longer because their symptoms are better managed. If you are still unsure, look into it and read some more. Arrange to visit a hospice before you become critically ill and talk to the staff.

The key message I want to leave you with is that entering palliative care is not a reflection of your coping ability, and nor does it in any way diminish you. On the contrary, it has the means to help you maximize your quality of life. It is most certainly worth considering.

Key Points

- Palliative-care services provide a range of vital support to cancer patients. They do not just tend dying patients.
- Early introduction to palliative-care supports can make a difference to your physical and psychological well-being due to better management and monitoring of your most troublesome symptoms.
- Palliative care mostly takes place in your own home although you may have the option of hospice-based care.
- Ask specifically for an introduction to palliative-care services if you feel you could benefit from them but your oncologist has not yet referred you.

28

How Do I Tell the Kids?

'Make sure you put in some advice about how to tell the kids,' a colleague urged me. My first response was, 'I don't know if I can. It's such a difficult topic.' 'You have to,' she insisted. 'You know how much our patients struggle with this. I know Karen does.'

I looked across at the row of chemotherapy chairs and realized to my dismay that nearly half of the patients receiving chemotherapy on that day were parents of young children. A forty-year-old patient named Karen caught my eye and smiled. Karen was a lovely woman, an actor. She had played good roles in local productions but her work had come to a sudden halt when she was diagnosed with cancer. Things looked good for many months, but lately she had become unwell and started another round of chemo. I had always been open with her, so she knew that this time my expectations of chemo were modest. She had decided she would give it a good try but if things were still not looking up after a few weeks, she would stop treatment and concentrate on being home with her three children, aged four, six and ten, and her husband, Jim.

I suspect there is no cancer patient and parent who doesn't fret about what and how to tell the children, but surprisingly, this is another topic rarely brought up in the consultation. Many patients don't feel it is a doctor's role to advise them on such personal matters, or imagine that they might be wasting their time discussing these issues when there are so many medical questions swirling in their mind.

I must also confess that most of my inquiries about the children of cancer patients go something like this:

'How are the kids doing?'

'Okay. Thank you for asking.'

'That's good to hear.'

As I write this I find myself reflecting that this desultory exchange is designed to protect both parent-patient and doctor from the awkwardness of discussing the single most difficult aspect of a serious illness – the dread of leaving young children behind.

Shortly after Karen sat down last week, I went through the checklist.

'And how are the children?'

'I'm really worried about them.'

'Tell me more,' I said, swallowing my apprehension.

'I will need your help in explaining things to them. I don't know where to start.'

Fearing that I would mess up the task, I promptly suggested the help of a skilled psychologist but Karen wasn't interested. 'I'm too tired, doctor. Plus, you're a mom, so you must have some idea about what to say to the kids. I just want you to guide me through it.' She looked at me with such hope that I promised to do my best.

Karen died two years after the date of her diagnosis. Her children were such an integral part of her life that we touched on them on nearly every occasion we met. Her devotion to her children's welfare, and by extension, the welfare of other similarly placed children, was so profound that I know she would be proud to let me share how we navigated each downward step in her journey. I hope Karen's story helps you navigate yours, if you are in this unenviable situation.

Karen's lung cancer was a bolt from the blue. She had never smoked, had no family history and was simply unlucky. When the diagnosis was confirmed, we also discussed that its spread meant that it was not curable. However, with several recent advances in treating her type of cancer, I was optimistic about keeping her well. Karen wanted to tell the children and overcame her husband Jim's early ambivalence.

She sat them down one evening and told them that she had been diagnosed with an illness called lung cancer. She deliberately chose to use the correct terminology rather than Jim's suggestion of calling it a lump. We had discussed the fact that children fell down in the playground and got lumps and bumps. She didn't want the children to think that all lumps were sinister. Their eldest, Alyssa, had seen the confronting ads depicting cancer on cigarette packets and her first question was if her mother had been smoking cigarettes. Karen and Jim had always pointed at the images as the consequences of smoking. Karen assured her daughter that she had never smoked and that sometimes people developed cancer for unknown reasons. Robbie, their middle son, wanted to know if she was going to die. He had a classmate who had just lost her grandfather to lung cancer. 'I'm not dying right now, darling', Karen told him. 'I hope to get better with treatment.' The youngest child, Emily, at four years old didn't understand any of the conversation. She jumped on her mother's back and chirped, 'Can we play hide-and-seek now?'

As she began chemotherapy, Karen decided to hope for the best and plan for the worst. She set about consolidating a support system for the children. She did this by calling upon a small group of parents whose children were friendly with hers. She told them openly what she knew – that she had lung cancer that was not curable. Her oncologist felt there was good treatment available but she was likely to become sicker with time. Karen told them that she had stopped working as she wanted to maximize her time with the children, but on the occasions when she was too unwell, she would need the parents' help. The parents, who were also Karen's friends, were shocked, but also felt proud to be asked to play a helping role.

Over the next few weeks, they worked out a system that meant that each child had one or two additional adults to rely on if Jim and Karen were both busy. On chemotherapy days, Emily was dropped off and picked up from kindergarten by her friend's mum. When Jim couldn't make it to Robbie's soccer practice, another father took him. Alyssa walked home to her friend's house after school and was later brought home by the friend's mother after the girls had finished their homework. When Karen felt well, which was almost always in the initial months, the extra help was not needed, but having a roster in place meant that the other adults were not surprised at being rung at short notice.

Jim's parents were frail and elderly and needed help themselves. But Karen's parents were able to assist. While they weren't able to drive the children back and forth from their activities, Karen's mother cooked healthy dinners and her dad helped with garden maintenance. Both offers freed up Karen and Jim to take care of other things.

A practical thing Karen discussed early with her children was rearranging after-school activities that required prolonged parental involvement. She explained to the children that while she was keen to maintain their activities, her illness meant that they all had to make some adjustments. For Alyssa this meant finding a French class closer to home rather than the one she had become used to, which was a five-hour weekend commitment. For Emily it meant moving a gymnastics class. Robbie offered to reduce the frequency of his painting lessons. Karen was initially apprehensive that she was asking too much of her children, to give up what they liked, but she soon realized that they felt proud to be helping their mum and gladly adjusted to their changes. Karen spoke to her children's school early in the piece too, letting them know about her diagnosis and the changes in their lives. The counsellor agreed to keep a close eye on all three and periodically provide updates to Karen and Jim.

One day Robbie came home, upset that a boy in his class had said he would catch cancer from his mum. On hearing this, Alyssa complained that she was sick of being asked if she was alright. Little Emily, meanwhile, carried on, seemingly oblivious to anything being out of the ordinary. Karen instinctively felt angry on behalf of her children, but used the occasion to discuss her cancer with them further. She reassured Robbie that cancer was not contagious and explained to Alyssa how much her friends and their parents cared about her. Karen also told them that her being sick was not the children's fault and that people sometimes said awkward things because they didn't know how to express their true feelings. Karen felt that this gave the children permission to discuss any other concerns they might have about her and bring home any comments they had heard on the playground. Sure enough, one day Robbie said to Jim, 'My friend said that cancer only happens to old people. Was he being mean to mum?' Jim was able to explain that cancer also happens to young people, but his friend was probably puzzled because he had not met anyone like that. Alyssa asked if her mum would lose all her hair like someone's aunty did and Karen reassured her that her therapy was different, so she would not.

Things went smoothly for nearly nine months and everyone fell into a comfortable pattern. One day, Karen came in for a quick visit with all three children, whom she left in the waiting room to watch TV when

I called her in. I asked how the children were doing and she replied that they were surprisingly normal. 'They watch my face and if I'm okay they are okay.'

Sadly, I won't forget that day because it was when I had to tell Karen that after more than a year of stability, the cancer had begun to spread to critical areas that concerned me. I also observed that she did not look as well as she had in the last few months. We talked about changing treatments and hoping for the best while expecting that treatments down the line would not work as well as the initial one. She listened worriedly and then burst into tears. 'Oh, what a bad day to bring the kids,' she said in a woeful understatement. Then I watched helplessly as she rose and washed her face in the sink, reapplied her lipstick, and said, 'We will handle it. I will talk to them.'

Some weeks later when we met again, I reluctantly asked how her talk had gone with her children. She said that directly after her consultation, she took them out for ice cream and enjoyed the occasion while suspending her fears. Later, with Jim present, she told the family that the cancer was becoming active again. She explained that she may feel some more pain but showed them the new tablets I had prescribed her to manage it. She mentioned the need to travel more frequently to hospital for the new treatment, but she would adjust her needs as far as possible to meet theirs. They needed to be prepared to have other adults assisting them more than usual. Karen talked seriously but kindly and slowly, telling the children that she wanted them to know the truth from her rather than hear snatches of conversations elsewhere that left them wondering what was going on. She told them that she would always be honest with them. This is when Alyssa asked if her mother was going to die.

'I will probably die one day from this cancer, but the doctor says it's not happening yet. So I plan to take the new treatment and be as well as possible, and I promise to let you know if things are not working out.' Karen said that this was the question she had been most dreading, but tackling it honestly had been far easier than offering excuses. Robbie had always been deeply perceptive. 'But Angie's grandma died in her sleep. What if that happens to you?' To this she replied, 'I suppose this could happen, but if I die in my sleep, you know that Daddy is healthy and perfectly able to look after you with the help of all our wonderful friends and family.' Karen said that since she could not reassure him about how or when she would die, she wanted to emphasize that they had a support structure in place that they had experienced and trusted. They would not be left alone.

As Karen began her new treatment, the children again settled into their routine and accepted a slightly different normality. Although it's easy to relate Karen's experiences here, I found it heart-wrenching to hear her accounts at the time. It seemed unfair that anyone, especially innocent children, should have to go through such grieving. But when I brought this up with Karen, she said with typical perspective, 'Doctor, it is what it is. I just want to prepare them for life without me and know that I have done my very best.' She also said that she was struck by how well the children took the news and how supportive they were. She observed, 'Sometimes I wonder why they're not sad or crying, but I know they understand the seriousness of it.'

For all but a month of the two years she had cancer, Karen avoided hospitalization. Her symptoms were remarkably few and always manageable. Although she slowed down significantly, she often sat in the car with Jim or a friend to see her children off to school and pick them up. She chatted to the school counsellor and was assured they were doing admirably well under the circumstances, which made her feel good.

The next big change came when she became very breathless and had to be hospitalized. Fluid was drained from one lung and she made a good recovery but was very tired. Emily visited her in hospital but her older children decided to wait for her at home. Karen sent them a message but didn't insist on their coming in, believing this was their way of coping and perhaps slowly coming to terms with her dying.

When Karen got home she again sat down with her children. She told them that a scan had shown things becoming worse, which matched how she was feeling. Alyssa asked if she was in a lot of pain and she truthfully answered she wasn't but the drugs she was taking made her drowsy. She told the kids not to mistake her drowsiness for disinterest. 'You know that seeing you always makes me happy.' Emily remained affectionate and playful but seemed to sense something was wrong.

She began to sit quietly with her mother and pat her hand or fetch a glass of water. Karen gave her daughter a lot of hugs and kept telling her how much she was loved. On one of her last visits, Karen told me that Robbie suddenly seemed distant and didn't want to talk about her illness even when asked. She worried that this meant he would struggle after her death, but Jim helped her realize that their son had always been quietly perceptive and strong. 'Robbie knows he can ask me anything, so I won't push him into any conversation.' I admired Karen and Jim's maturity and ability to view things from their children's perspective.

Soon after this, Karen was admitted to a hospice one day when the children were at school. She was too weak to remain at home and needed assistance with activities including toileting and feeding. But her mind remained alert. I visited her there and she asked me how long she had. It was a distressing exchange for us both but I told her that I thought time was very short.

That evening the children visited her in the hospice. Jim had explained where she was and what to expect. He showed them pictures of her oxygen tubing and her room. He agreed with Alyssa that their mum looked gaunt and not like the mum they had even a few months ago. He told Emily that her mum was sick and was going to meet God. Robbie asked if it was going to be quick and Jim said the doctor expected it to be, but it would relieve mum of more suffering because the cancer could not be cured.

On Karen's suggestion, Jim gave the children a choice. He said they could see their mum on Skype or FaceTime or visit her in the hospice. He told them their mum understood this might make them sad and she was proud of what they had put up with so far. Alyssa and Emily wanted to go but Robbie wasn't sure, so Jim took the girls. Karen greeted her daughters with a smile and told her she was comfortable. She introduced them to her nurse, who praised their mum and told them how proud Karen was of them. The girls beamed at the compliment. Emily looked around curiously and was delighted to notice some of her pictures stuck to the wall.

Alyssa later told Robbie that she had felt nervous earlier because she had feared her mum would be crying but seeing her comfortable made her happy. This gave Robbie the strength to go in later himself. He was greeted similarly by his mum who also told him that it was okay to feel odd being there and he didn't have to stay. This gave Robbie permission to ask his dad soon afterwards to take him home. Emily came every day but mainly played with the toys outside.

In the hospice a volunteer had asked Karen whether she wanted to dictate or film a memento for her children. Karen started cautiously but became too distressed to continue. She told me that she felt she had shared enough with her children in the past two years and that she was happy they would remember her. I held her hand and agreed.

Four days later, Karen became unconscious. She was sedated and looked peaceful. Jim was devastated but true to Karen's promise, kept the children involved till the end. They all came to visit and expressed a wish to remain there. 'Mom always looked after us, now it's our turn to stay with her.' Jim asked the nurse whether this would harm the children psychologically, but she assured him that she had seen other children present at a parent's death. The priest arrived and they prayed together. One after the other, they all said goodbye to Karen. When the older children cried, Emily copied them. Jim just held them and reassured them he would look after them. All the grandparents arrived in time to watch Karen breathe her last.

Some months later, Jim dropped by to say thank you to the staff. Naturally, I asked about the children. He said that they were sad but appropriately so. They were continuing with their activities and talked about their mom when they wanted. They talked to her too. Every night they told their mom about something that had happened during the day. He encouraged this, and in fact, liked to tell them that she would be proud. 'They ask me if I miss her terribly and I say I do, but she would like us all to go on being happy. I think they worry about being disloyal to her memory and I tell them that she will always be their mom.'

Jim admitted that he had been initially unsure about 'letting the kids in', but Karen convinced him that it was best to be honest and sensitive with them for long-term benefit. He had feared they were being burdened but realized now that being involved at an age-appropriate level was the best way forward. Jim now belongs to a parent-support group, where he counsels other parents about talking to children about cancer.

When Karen first asked me to help I was anxious because I scarcely knew what the best advice was. I don't think she needed my help. In turns, I was struck, saddened and humbled by the decisive way in which she dealt with her blow. She also left me with a meaningful prototype for advising future patients who ask the same question and I no longer feel as apprehensive discussing the matter. I can't help thinking that Karen would be surprised but quietly delighted at her legacy.

Key Points

- Sharing a life-threatening diagnosis with children is one of the most difficult things you will do.
- Plan ahead and don't hesitate to seek assistance from all those who are willing.
- Use all the help necessary to minimize disruption to children's routine but know that children are resilient and will adapt to changes around them.
- Decide on what is age-appropriate information but also follow your instincts. Children's curiosity and desire for information and engagement evolve and fluctuate with time.
- You will not always be stoic and it's okay, indeed normal, for children to witness and experience emotion.
- Not everyone wants to leave behind a written or recorded legacy, but palliative-care services can assist with this if you do.

29

Keeping Hope Alive

In consultation with a patient, Bob, I begin in my usual manner to ascertain what the patient knows about his diagnosis.

'Tell me what you have found out so far,' I ask him.

I suspect from his drawn face that he hasn't slept much lately. He looks at his wife, Mary, wearily and then at me, with a slightly curious expression, as if to say, 'Aren't you the one who should be telling me things?'

I quickly explain that although I have his history at hand, it helps me to hear about his condition in his own words. He starts haltingly: 'Six weeks ago I started feeling pain and saw my doctor, who discovered a tumour in my pancreas. He sent me to a surgeon who organized more tests before telling me that he couldn't remove it safely. He thought I should see you for chemo.'

Mary adds: 'The surgeon also said that if Bob had a really good response to chemotherapy he would have another look at performing an operation. He was happy with Bob's fitness level.'

'That's a really good summary,' I say. 'Now tell me a little bit about yourself.'

Bob is forty-five-years-old. Mary is his second wife. His first marriage broke down six years ago when his wife left him for a work colleague. After two years of court battles, Bob has won partial custody of his two children from that marriage. The twin girls are ten years old and seem to be doing well emotionally after a tumultuous early childhood. He hasn't shared his news with them yet.

'I kept blaming my pain on the stress from the custody matter but clearly there was something else going on,' he sighs.

'Pancreatic cancer almost always creeps up on people,' I say, sympathetically. 'You behaved like most other young and fit people would in your circumstances.'

'Maybe it could have been removed earlier,' he ventures.

'Judging by its position, I doubt it,' I tell him.

'But there are things you can do, right?'

'Yes, we can treat it.'

'So he can be cured,' Mary states.

'About that, I'm not sure, especially at this early stage when you haven't yet had any treatment.'

'So what will treatment achieve if you can't cure me?' I can see Bob is already disappointed at my remark.

'Treatment means keeping the tumour under control, stopping it from growing and preventing it from causing pain and other complications.'

'So is there, what, a fifty-fifty chance of cure?'

'Bob, the scan shows a fairly large tumour with involved lymph glands. I'm going to give you the best treatment possible but I would hesitate to say that the chance of a complete cure is high as that.'

'I'm dying,' he says, morosely.

'Your life is not under immediate threat,' I respond gently. 'Let's give chemo a chance.'

'Darling, let's do that,' Mary adds. 'Take one thing at a time.'

Bob's eyes are glimmering with tears. 'Doctor, you're my only hope. Stay with me on this one.'

I hear these words often and they confer a humbling faith in my abilities but also an enormous responsibility. Keep me well, the patient says. And also keep my hope alive.

Every oncologist wants to protect patients from harm and help them live longer. We also see the practical value of having hope – it smooths the journey for both patient and doctor when there is something to look forward to. Everyone talks about patients who lost hope and then died – although this is not necessarily true every time, it is an evocative concept with which we all identify. We do need something to live for.

But before I discuss hope, I want to say that if you are feeling hopeless about your situation, you are experiencing a normal emotion.

If you are depressed, there is help. And if you are very unwell, it is not your hopelessness but the disease process that has got you there, so please don't be hard on yourself. And if you are a worried carer, it helps to remember that you can't persuade somebody to discover hope, but your gentle support can make a difference.

It's no wonder that oncologists, being only human, feel a keenness to maintain and even fuel hope in their patients. It is admittedly easier to nourish hope when things are going well, in which case a kind word or a simple reassurance is enough to restore a patient's transiently diminished spirits. For example, a patient who is on the verge of finishing chemotherapy can be reassured that many of his worst side effects will subside. Someone who is upset about never being able to have children can be shown the favourable statistics that say otherwise.

Before going on to discussing hope when things are genuinely not faring well, I want to turn to the important role that a spouse, carer, close friends and family can play in keeping hope alive. Hope is not only a function of a patient's medical status but is derived from many other things including how much respect, dignity and empathy someone senses from those close to him. 'Our extended family has always met for Sunday lunch. Now, when I am no longer well and able to go out, I love that everyone still gets together as if nothing has changed. Sometimes, I am too tired to last the entire afternoon but it always buoys me to see them. Frankly, they give me hope.'

Sometimes families and friends withdraw from a patient in a wish to allow you space. They may not know how to best support you. If this sounds familiar, you might want to reassure them that their company is enough. Sharing other people's news and staying connected to the outside world nourish many spirits. When others ask me about the best way to help a cancer patient, I often advise, 'Sit with them and you will find out.'

Let me return now to the role of the oncologist in keeping hope alive. Even when the odds don't look good it's difficult to look a patient in the eye and say so; it's easier to play for time or nudge patients along on morsels of hope. In the back of every oncologist's mind are the anecdotes of patients who have defied terrible prognoses and lived to tell the tale. It is mortifying to tell a patient that he has three or six months left and find out that you were wrong. Even if a doctor gets prognosis roughly correct on many occasions, it takes just one or two mistaken ones to become cautious about future frank conversations.

However, research repeatedly tells us that patients want their oncologist to tell them the truth, even if they are dying. Different patients may want to know varying degrees of information but no one wants to be kept in the dark. How to maintain hope while telling the truth is one of the thorniest dilemmas of being an oncologist.

What I have learnt from my patients is that attempts to hide the truth, or ignore informed instincts about the patient, usually backfire. It can mean patients who wrongly believed that they were permanently cured learn that this was never so. Or those who endure gruelling months of chemotherapy find out that there was only ever a modest chance of the cancer shrinking, let alone being cured. Patients who kept putting off their long-planned holiday until they ended treatment discover that it will be actually indefinite. Those who believe that the oncologist would tell them when further treatment is futile feel betrayed when they discover they never had a chance to come off it.

You will hear plenty of disillusioned patients assert that they were sold false hope. A troubling situation is when patients with advanced cancer rue that their prognosis was either wildly exaggerated or in fact never discussed, thus robbing them of the opportunity to attend to some important tasks. A patient recently said, 'The doctor kept saying things were okay and there was another chemo to try if this one failed. But I wish she had told me the truth that nothing was working the way we expected. Now I am too sick to travel. I regret the wasted time.'

I later ran into this patient's doctor at a conference and we talked about him.

'He wanted to live so badly that I felt terrible disappointing him. So I kept coming up with ideas, but at the bottom of my heart, I knew that he wasn't going to do well. I tried to hint at it, but I felt as if he wasn't listening. Finally, I just had to say I had tried enough times and I'd wait for him.'

As a patient you are probably wondering how the oncologist could conceal such vital information from the patient. If you are a doctor you are nodding because this situation happens all too commonly,

A mismatch of perceptions and the reluctance to open up difficult conversations means that things are postponed for another day, or maybe for another doctor to broach.

A colleague described her grandfather's experience like this: 'His oncologist spends all the time looking at tests. Grandpa is eighty-five and frail – he needs to hear that he is incurable because he keeps making plans that are years away. But the oncologist refuses to see the forest for the trees, and when we come home, Grandpa says he's doing fine because the doctor didn't say any different. It's exasperating and sad for the family.'

On another occasion, a devoted carer said of her ill uncle: 'I know it's difficult but I'd love his oncologist to somehow tell him he is dying but also give him hope for the life still left. He relies on his doctors for hope.'

Hope is important in our lives. Hope nourishes us and infuses meaning into whatever trouble we endure. When you first heard you had cancer you naturally hoped that it wasn't the case. Then you hoped it was curable. If you heard it was not curable, you hoped that chemotherapy would be a good fix. When the first chemotherapy fails, you hope that the second one won't. There is always the hope of new discoveries, clinical trials and a miracle.

It is true of doctors too. When I first meet a patient, it's my greatest hope that their cancer is curable. When treatment falters, there is usually room to try something else and hope that works. When the patient does not look well, I hope that the setback is temporary. When the patient asks for a prognosis, I often say that I hope I am wrong and that the patient outlives my expectations. I come to work every day hoping that I can keep all my patients well – hope fuels my actions.

Both doctor and patient derive solace from hope. But hope is different from wishful thinking. There is absolutely nothing wrong with hoping that you will get better or that you will be cured, but it is important to be prepared for worse. You can probably think of other life experiences where this has been true. You hope that you will be the successful job applicant but have a Plan B. You hope that yours will be the winning bid on a new house but prepare to try elsewhere if the price goes too high. As human beings we have the capacity to hope as well as the resilience to tackle disappointment.

Maintaining hope is certainly important but don't rely on it overly to help you live longer or better. Instead, I would suggest framing your hope on honest reality to help you make good decisions about your health. I want to show you how this is possible.

Begin by really understanding what the goals of care are in your case. As we've discussed, cancer patients receive care for many reasons. Cure is one but where cure is not possible, the goal may be to shrink the cancer, prevent further growth, avoid complications, prevent pain and discomfort, and live better. Remembering that goals change, talk to your oncologist periodically about which of these to expect so that there is no room for a vital misconception.

One of the many memorably upsetting moments for me as an oncologist was when I met a lady with advanced cancer for the first time. She had developed spinal cord compression and couldn't feel her legs or walk. I heard that she had failed several lines of chemotherapy and had been thinking of enrolling in a clinical trial before this new problem occurred. I told her that we could treat the spinal problem with radiotherapy but while her back pain might improve, I was not confident that she would return to walking. I also prescribed proper analgesia. Then, with her husband listening, she asked if she would live to Christmas. It was June.

'Tell me why you want to know and I will answer the question to the best of my ability,' I said.

'My son is going to propose to his girlfriend at the Christmas table and I wouldn't want to miss it.'

I knew that she already had a poor prognosis because of the heavy burden of disease. The spinal cord compression was an added impairment that would severely limit her mobility and make her vulnerable to infections and other complications. Having treated many patients like her, my estimation was that she had only weeks to live.

Trying to decide how to tell her, I explored further. 'What do you think about your condition?'

'Well, this is a setback but I am strong and I am going to beat this. I will be cured one day.'

I began by telling her that estimations of prognosis can be incorrect but I wanted to give her some kind of answer that would be helpful.

After some more explanation, this is how I finished: 'So, unfortunately, I think that you may be quite ill towards Christmas and there is a chance you may not make it. If being at your son's proposal is very important to you, I would suggest sharing this news with him and seeing whether he might want to propose earlier.'

The patient burst into tears at the news. She said she had no idea about the gravity of her situation and her husband looked equally shocked. We spoke at great length and by the time I left she felt genuinely grateful for my advice, saying that it had made her shift her priorities. I felt sad but relieved that the conversation had gone well.

But by the next morning, she was extremely angry with me. The reason was that her first oncologist who saw her at diagnosis sixteen months ago had told her that she had at least five years to live. Following our talk, she tracked down that oncologist who was non-committal because he hadn't seen her for many months. He couldn't come to see her but balked at the idea that he'd given her a good prognosis. 'It's clear she had terrible biology from the start but she never asked how long,' he told me when I got in touch. The distressed patient remained in hospital due to continued complications and died just two weeks after our chat. Everyone who met her remarked on her anger and disillusionment at the mixed messages she had received. But in fact, she had perceived two messages – two different appraisals from different doctors. One, that she would live many years and another, that she didn't have long. It's the fact that the difference in the two estimates was so vast and ominous that she couldn't get over her shock. I thought I was trying to make her final days meaningful; she accused me of crushing her hope.

Be clear in your mind about the goals of your care. Write them down in your doctor's office if you need. And remember that goals can change, so it makes sense to review them from time to time. For example, the initial goal may have been to shrink the tumour, but if you have since had the tumour removed, is a cure now feasible? Conversely, your treatment may have been given with the intent to cure, but if you didn't respond to the treatment, has the goal changed to keeping the cancer in one place for as long as possible? Doctors can slip into medical jargon such as progressive disease, remission, stable disease and overall survival in describing your condition. It's important that you understand what these terms mean in plain language. Don't guess or promise to read up on it later. Ask the person using these terms what they mean in your context.

Negotiate with your doctor how you will discuss important milestones in your treatment. Do you want to look at your X-rays, keep copies of your report and explore all the details, or are you someone who prefers broader brushstrokes of information? Either way, if you are after the truth, explicitly say so to your doctor: 'No matter what, I would like you to be honest with me about my cancer.' Doctors don't set out to be dishonest with their patients, but hearing a clear message that the patient wants to be a partner in their treatment, and is not afraid to hear bad news, makes it more likely that your oncologist will be open with you. And if the doctor has to then deliver bad news, you need to remind yourself that this was part of your pact. I can't help thinking that the patient with spinal cord compression described above would have benefited from such a pact that allowed her to discover information slowly and in her own time.

If the goals of care are clear in your own mind and you can talk to your oncologist honestly and freely about a change in circumstances, you are in a better place than most – you are empowered. The truth is that nobody can guarantee you will always be well. However, there are many people who will help you live well in the present. Time and again I see that the patients who come to terms with uncertainty are the ones who live life well.

In the months following our initial meeting, as Bob realized that his cancer was not curable, he felt despondent and expressed a wish to die sooner rather than prolonging the inevitable. I asked him to give himself time. Sure enough, the initial shock dissipated and with the help of his wife Mary and his parents he could see that he was still well and able to do things. He started chemotherapy and between cycles focused on readying a new, larger room for his twins. A skilled woodworker, he enjoyed making them a beautiful desk. He couldn't believe it when it was finished, confessing he feared he wouldn't live to see it. He quickly moved on to crafting chairs.

The couple had a beach house where the family now made it a point to go on weekends. Bob found the wide expanse of water relaxing and eventually decided to return to fishing, a keen hobby he had let lapse. He was delighted to find he was still good at it. 'I never thought that a cancer patient would have the stamina to go out in a boat!' he exclaimed.

Bob kept discovering that he could do the things he enjoyed, provided he thought them through and paced himself. Once he learned to savour the present, he found his worries eased. 'Some call it living with cancer. I call it living around cancer. There are days when I feel sad or worried and I don't fight them. They pass and I think of the desk that I made or a beautiful morning on the water, and I am grateful.'

Bob remained fit for longer than expected, surprising everyone including himself. I believe that part of his wellness came from adapting to change. When he became weak, he gave up woodcutting but began instructing an apprentice. When he could no longer fish, he sat at the edge of the water, letting the waves lap at his feet. When he became frail, he said he was proud of using his time well. 'I feel that I was a good role model to my girls.'

After he passed away, his wife observed that she could not believe the transformation in him during his illness. She said that keeping small goals in sight had made such a difference in his life that she had fewer regrets now that he was no more.

Bob lost hope, then found it again, in small, everyday things.

Key Points

- Sustaining hope is important but guard against false hope, which might eventually let you down.
- Being clear about your goals of care at all stages of an illness helps you handle serious discussions without losing hope.
- Negotiate with your oncologist how you might address important milestones. Outline how much information you desire and whom you might want to include in those discussions.
- Honest discussions with your oncologist might well involve discussing bad news. Think about how you will handle them.

30

Advance-Care Planning

Seventy-year-old Mrs Formosa was receiving treatment for advanced oral cancer. Two years ago, surgery and radiotherapy left her with cosmetic and functional defects. Her mouth didn't close properly, leaving a slight gap on one side through which food and saliva constantly leaked. The leakage led to chronic low-grade inflammation of the surrounding facial skin,which became periodically infected, at which time she would stop chemotherapy and begin treatment with antibiotics. She continued like this for many months, thanks in large part to her determination.

The altered anatomy of Mrs Formosa's head and neck was so complex that even experts found it hard to interpret her scans. At best, the scans looked no worse and there was no evident progression of disease. When scans are not greatly helpful, some doctors use symptoms to gauge the value of treatment. But here too, her chronic complaint that she was embarrassed by the leakage from her mouth got no better with time. Although she was not suffering from severe side effects of chemotherapy, she had no quality of life either, nothing changed. It seemed on some days that we were on a journey without strong meaning.

One afternoon Mrs Formosa became severely short of breath. Her husband called an ambulance and the paramedics correctly diagnosed her as suffering from aspiration pneumonia, caused by food entering the lungs due to impaired swallowing. She was admitted to a hospital ward but deteriorated overnight. When it appeared that she would need intensive care, a call was made to the family about her wishes regarding aggressive treatment in the presence of advanced cancer. The family was bewildered, admitting that they had never foreseen this situation. They had always assumed that she would fade away slowly at home. In desperation, her husband wanted to talk to each of their six children for advice but since there was no time to waste, Mrs Formosa ended up being intubated and placed on a ventilator.

Once she was in intensive care, the family decided to see whether Mrs Formosa made any progress. Four days later, her pneumonia looked worse and her organs were failing. The family urged the doctors to do more. Artificial feeding and temporary dialysis were commenced, but to no avail. The family felt upset by the escalating intervention which wasn't making her better. But being deeply religious, they didn't feel they could sanction withdrawal of care. The intensive-care doctors were conflicted but felt that the patient's life was being unnecessarily and painfully prolonged. Mrs Formosa continued to deteriorate and died after a few more days. Her family was traumatized by the whole episode and couldn't believe this is how her life ended.

Contrast this to the family of Mr Giles, a man of similar age with a perforated bowel cancer. The perforation led to severe infection and cardiac strain exacerbated by two previous heart attacks. Unconscious, Mr Giles was admitted to intensive care for stabilization. The surgeon advised the family that he could attempt an operation but he seriously doubted Mr Giles's ability to survive. Even if he did survive, the chances of meaningful recovery were dismal. However, the dilemma was that without surgery the patient was certain to die. Upon hearing this, his wife spoke up: 'He swore never to have surgery again after his first operation two years ago for cancer. He said he would die rather than go under the knife again.' All his assembled children nodded in agreement, recalling his vehement opposition to surgery because of the pain and debility he had experienced.

A unanimous decision was made to not operate but also to institute palliative care, which meant that Mr Giles was transferred out of the intensive care unit into a single room with appropriate pain relief and sedation. He was never ventilated and didn't receive any aggressive intervention. His family sat with him and watched him die peacefully within one day. They all said that although saddened by his untimely death they felt comfortable that they had respected his wishes. 'We used to tell Dad to stop being so morose, but we were so grateful that he was vocal about his wishes. He made our decisions straightforward.'

The difference between Mrs Formosa and Mr Giles was that he had clearly articulated his view about the direction of future care to the people his doctors turned to for guidance. I was reminded once again about the importance of having an advance care directive and I would like to talk you through what this means.

Advance care planning refers to a set of steps that you, as the patient, should take in order to ensure that your health care providers are clear about your wishes regarding your medical care. These instructions give you a voice in decision making even when you are sick or confused, or for some other reason unable to communicate effectively with your doctors at the time of an event.

Far too many people think only in terms of the present. When they feel energetic and well, or when their doctor gives them good news about successful cancer treatment, they cannot imagine that one day there may be serious issues to contend with. Or if such issues present themselves, many find it unimaginable that they may not be able to deal with them with a clear mind.

If you are feeling well right now, I challenge you to imagine being in Mrs Formosa's place. Can you picture yourself hooked up to a ventilator, multiple machines and IV lines, sedated and unconscious? Imagine your anxious spouse, children or grandchildren summoned to a meeting where they are asked if you ever expressed any clear wishes about how you might want to be treated. The vast majority of families say that the issue was never raised because discussing it seemed too close for comfort. 'I didn't want to jinx his recovery or dampen his spirits by asking him what he wanted at the end of life,' one wife reflected tearfully. 'But now I wish I had because I don't want to carry the burden alone.'

Some families that have the courage to broach the matter say that the discussion was usually brief and without any outcome. As one man remarked, when caught in a bind about deciding how to deal with his mother's all-too-plain suffering in the intensive care unit (ICU), 'When Grandma was in ICU, Mom kept saying, "I wouldn't want to go like that", but she was also the one who fought the hardest to keep Grandma there because she couldn't bear to let go.'

As an oncologist, I accompany many patients on their journey from diagnosis through to palliative care and eventual death. For some the journey is smooth because at each step they are able to clarify their wishes in order for me to institute appropriate management. For example, a patient who has previously rejected palliative-care nurses visiting his home recognizes that his escalating needs cannot be managed by reporting to the emergency department every week, and finally accepts the referral. Palliative care is instituted and his wife is relieved. Or a patient who has always insisted on receiving chemotherapy appreciates the steady decline in her condition and finally says she has had enough. She goes back to her residential care where her family doctor periodically visits her and she dies peacefully. What happened to both these patients would probably have happened anyway, but their ability to express their wishes and participate in the negotiations meant that things happened with their consent. They felt like partners in their care rather than passive recipients of external decision making.

At a time when many people feel vulnerable and upset, retaining these important aspects of decision-making capacity makes a great difference. It is a regrettable experience for everyone when it is evident that the patient is on a steep downward slope but there is no consensus on letting go. The word 'denial' is tossed around at these times, applied both to the patient and carers but it strikes me that it isn't denial so much as fear of the unknown that lets people either make poor decisions about their care or no decision at all.

Advance care planning refers to the act of thinking through your wishes for health care in the event you become seriously unwell or are dying. Your wishes should be ideally written down in a document or at the very least, conveyed to those who are closest to you and may be expected to make important health care decisions on your behalf. If you live in a region where your spoken intent is not enough, you must make sure that your wishes are properly documented and meet legal requirements. This may be unusual in the Indian context, but this doesn't mean you shouldn't consider it.

In the next section I want to help you think through advance care planning. The first step is to understand your illness and its prognosis, remembering that unexpected things can still happen. Advise your oncologist that you are thinking about advance care planning so that any information he provides can be tailored to future needs. Discuss the likely ways in which you could deteriorate but also include sudden, catastrophic things that could go wrong. What treatment might be offered in each instance and how effective would it be in reversing the situation? What sort of side effects might you expect from any treatment? For example, if your lung cancer suddenly began bleeding, what are the different things doctors might try to stop it? Would there be invasive procedures? What would be the chances of coming off a ventilator successfully if you were intubated in an emergency situation? If a cancer gets perforated, that is burst, what would happen with or without an operation? What might your quality of life look like after emergency surgery? You may not get clear answers, and every doctor has a different comfort level for engaging these admittedly difficult questions, but articulating them also helps you to think about your own views.

The next step is to use information about your cancer and its prognosis to define goals of care. It is possible that with the answers you receive to the above questions about a bleeding lung cancer, you decide you would never accept intervention and would rather be kept comfortable and sedated. Or you might decide that you would want to give interventions one try but not repeat them. After hearing about emergency abdominal surgery you might decide that your odds would not be favourable to even attempt a procedure, even if it were technically feasible. You can see that your own philosophy plays an important role here.

Take another example. The radiation oncologist tells you that you have spinal cord compression at multiple levels, which explains your recent inability to walk and the loss of control over bowel and bladder function. You are advised that surgery is not possible, and because the symptoms have appeared over some weeks, it's unlikely that radiotherapy will help you walk again. Although radiotherapy will not prolong life and you are unlikely to avoid being in a wheelchair, she is willing to treat you, hoping at best, to alleviate discomfort. You calculate that you would rather not spend three hours a day making the return trip to radiotherapy for limited or no gain. You would rather be in a wheelchair, accept a urinary catheter for hygiene, choose good pain relief, and spend the remainder of your life in your house that overlooks the mountains. You have actively used the information available to you to make a decision about how you want to spend the rest of your life. Even if the outcome is grave, patients describe being at peace when they feel involved in their care.

You may know exactly what you want to do about your future health and see it absolutely clearly in your mind's eye. You may always have known that you hate injections and prefer patches, that you prefer to be asleep and sedated than awake and distressed, that you would never ever enter the intensive care unit again, that you have a strong objection to receiving artificial feeding, or that your greatest dread is being dehydrated. But if nobody knows your views they are unlikely to be heeded, despite the best intention of those around you. I know that no doctor or nurse sets out to actively disrespect a patient's wishes, but the most common reason patients receive futile care or care against their desire is that no one is familiar with the patient's wishes, in which case it seems safer to do everything than be more selective.

Some people fear that by expressing instructions that they want a certain type of care they will put themselves in a bind, but this is not true. Your instructions to doctors can change – the key is to have given some thought to them.

Of course you may only have one or two things that really matter to you – for example, you do not wish to receive any further blood transfusions or you are not prepared to undergo more surgery. Having your wishes in writing is always a good idea. If possible, use an approved form, if your state or territory has one. Other signatures, such as that of an approved witness or your doctor, may be required. It's a good idea to ensure that the people most closely involved in your care, medical and personal, are aware of the document and have a copy of it. If you regularly attend a particular hospital or live in a residential facility, ask for a copy to be kept in the medical records. Since records are often not easily transferrable or accessible in an emergency, it's important that you or someone close to you keeps a copy ready for use.

Some patients fear that their wishes may not be respected because of legal loopholes, but in my experience doctors and families are almost uniformly relieved to have directions from the patient about future care. Concern about having a foolproof document should not be an excuse for not preparing one at all. If in doubt, there are professionals who can help you fill out some simple paperwork – just ask your doctor or nurse.

Despite understanding the importance of advance care planning, some people find they just cannot write down their wishes because they can't bear its finality. If you feel like this, you can appoint someone to make decisions on your behalf by keeping your interests in mind. This role has a formal title, variously called medical power of attorney, medical agent, enduring power of attorney or medical guardian. Remember that this person is supposed to act in your best interest. In other words, he or she should be able to express to the doctor what *you* would want and not what *they* desire should happen. When emotion is high, this role requires objectivity, so you should think carefully about who the best person may be to represent your interests. It may not necessarily be one of your children or your spouse – it may well be your friend or a colleague. As far as possible, ensure that others are aware of whom you have nominated. Communicating clearly with your family when you are well reduces the chances that there will be disagreement about the direction of your care. Importantly, it also removes a difficult burden from the shoulders of your family and loved ones who may not know what is right for you. Nominating a medical power of attorney doesn't mean that you sign away your rights to express your wishes or change your mind. As long as you are competent, your doctors will turn to you for decision making. The medical power of attorney is activated when you are not able to make decisions.

Many people find that their viewpoint changes with changing circumstances. You may have previously rejected an intervention that you now feel might help you. Or you may have decided that something you were previously keen to have is no longer in your best interest. By reviewing your advance care directive periodically, as well as the role of others who act as your agent, you can ensure that any documents reflect your present view.

Again, the time to make an advance care directive is when you are well and can think clearly about your options. In advanced cancer, the influence of fatigue, multiple medications and greater vulnerability, amongst other factors, may diminish your capacity to engage more fully in this important task. It may seem confronting, but in an era when it seems increasingly easy to prolong futile care, you and your family will be thankful that you did it.

Key Points

- An advance care directive is a document that sets out your goals of care during the last days of your life, especially in terms of which interventions you may or may not wish to have. It is important that you articulate your wishes when you are still able to contemplate them.
- It is becoming increasingly valuable to have an advance care directive in order to avoid futile and painful care during your last days.
- Families are very grateful to have a critically ill patient's own wishes guiding them at a time of high emotion.
- Your oncologist and a variety of other professionals can help you formulate an advance care directive.

31

Will My Death Be Painful?

Over the course of their illness, many cancer patients must come to terms with eventually dying from the disease. While this is usually acknowledged, there is a common fear about it that is rarely discussed. It is the question of *how* cancer sufferers die. Almost everyone seems to want to know but nobody knows quite how to ask this awkward question. Sometimes patients fear that asking is inviting the worst upon themselves. Relatives would often like to be better prepared but find it hard to contemplate someone's final phase of life without knowing what to expect.

If you are coming to terms with terminal cancer, I hope that your oncologist has clarified any questions about prognosis and that you are linked in to appropriate palliative care. It is then valuable to consider what happens next. As one patient recently told me, 'I know I'm dying, but I'm curious to know how it will happen. I think it will help me relax.' Feeling self-conscious, he then asked, 'Does that sound weird to you?'

I told him I thought it was a good question. Death in cancer patients can take a few forms. Many patients will notice a step-by-step deterioration in their condition, meaning that they are unable to do the things that were previously easy. This may range from tidying the house or driving locally to fixing a sandwich or walking to the bathroom independently. There may be days when a normal routine is possible followed by other days when it's not.

While some people can remain very well up to their final days, for most, fatigue is prominent. You might find that you need a prolonged period of rest between short bursts of activity. This can be frustrating and many patients describe such intense fatigue that it becomes difficult to contemplate performing even those activities that were once pleasurable. Long periods of time may be spent resting but true restfulness may still feel elusive. Gradually, you may not feel like getting out of bed at all, but might still enjoy seeing people for short periods. Slowly, the exertion of conversation may feel too much and interest in food and drink wanes.

From spending more time resting or sleeping, many people drift into periods of reduced consciousness. Contrary to what people fear, patients can still have lucid breaks when they recognize familiar faces and are able to express likes and dislikes; for example, a particular food or a special friend. While most patients are not able to consume full meals by this time, they may eat a spoonful of ice cream, swallow some soup or ask for a drink. As we've discussed, it's particularly difficult for families to watch a loved one lose all interest in food, and almost everyone fears that lack of nutrition and hydration will hasten death. But it's important to understand that the lack of interest in engaging with people or having food and drink is normal – it's very much a part of the dying process. In some cases, oral intake may precipitate pain, nausea or vomiting, understandably causing greater reluctance to eat.

Severe anaemia can lead to death. In terminal conditions, a blood transfusion often doesn't help symptoms, leading patients to decide that they will no longer have their blood tests monitored or have a transfusion. Periods of reduced consciousness slowly merge into unconsciousness. Many patients become peacefully unconscious, although others may display outward signs of agitation. They can appear restless and twitchy while some may groan periodically or call out. A number of factors contribute to agitation. Although not everyone experiences pain, nausea or physical discomfort, it is a possible cause of agitation. Fear, anxiety or a desire to hold out to see a loved one may also play a role, and this is hopefully recognized with close observation and, if appropriate, gentle questioning. When none of these factors is readily identifiable, or they have been adequately treated, it is possible that proteins secreted by the cancer are contributing to agitation and confusion.

Theoretically, patients have a multitude of reasons to be uncomfortable and it can be difficult for doctors and loved ones to figure out exactly which symptom is responsible for how much discomfort or agitation. But towards the end of life, what matters most is being able to ensure comfort regardless of the precise contribution of each problem. Depending on the level of services involved, patients may need medical and palliative-care assistance to render them comfortable. It is unsafe to swallow tablets or capsules if a patient is not fully alert, but alternative means such as patches, injections and syringe drivers that continuously deliver medicines through the skin are available through good palliative-care services. Unfortunately, for many people, palliative care remains a vague concept, but things are changing slowly as we discover the importance of good end-of-life care, not just for the patient but also for surviving relatives, who report better emotional health. Many patients who suffer more from existential distress than physical can have these issues dealt with by expert professionals too.

Not everyone needs a palliative-care specialist to manage end-of-life care, and indeed, most patients get by with the help of a caring family and an involved family doctor. Where available, community and palliative-care nurses play a critical role in ensuring patient comfort. Where such infrastructure doesn't exist, doctors and community hospitals have been successfully able to teach family members some basic care skills.

Usually, an unconscious patient's breathing will slow down notably, and towards the end, become infrequent, before death occurs. If you have been watching over someone you will notice a change in breathing. Some patients are heard to sigh before taking a final breath while others simply fail to take another breath. A changed or mottled appearance of the hands and feet may be apparent as less oxygen enters the bloodstream and the circulation becomes sluggish.

One of the most frustrating things for loved ones who maintain a vigil by an unconscious patient's bedside is predicting when the patient will die. Naturally, relatives always stress that they are not eager for the person to die but wish the painful journey to end for their loved one's sake. Far from being unkind, it is a reasonable and practical question to ask, especially in an ageing society where an elderly and often unwell spouse doesn't possess the stamina to remain by the bedside day and night, despite good intentions.

Modern medicine can predict many more things than it used to, but it is still difficult to say just when an unconscious patient will die. Some patients seem to hang on for days while others deteriorate rather quickly. Sometimes the deterioration is obvious and its course predictable, other times it's not. Sometimes, if a cancer patient has other serious illnesses, such as heart or lung disease or organ failure, the combination of illnesses can extract a greater toll, whereas if cancer is the only major illness, and the patient is young, it may take time for the body to wind down. In essence, predicting death remains an inexact science. However, an experienced doctor should be able to indicate whether death is expected broadly within hours, days or longer. Bear in mind, however, that even the most experienced doctors can get predictions incorrect. Before you brand this a failing of the medical profession, consider that it's a reflection of human biology, not medical expertise.

Regrettably, despite everyone's best intentions, there are cancer deaths that are not orderly, peaceful or predictable. Catastrophes such as uncontrolled bleeding, deep vein thrombosis, uncontrolled pain and unrelenting depression do happen, both from cancer and its treatment. Cancer doesn't occur to the exclusion of other illnesses, and fatal heart attacks, strokes or other events also affect patients. In the quest to tackle cancer, the management of other conditions takes a back seat, which can sometimes lead to complications. In other words, much like so many aspects of life, it isn't possible for every step of the cancer experience to be planned.

If palliative-care professionals are involved with a patient at home, they may suggest to the family to keep so-called *catastrophic medications* at hand to relieve any evident suffering. Many family members resort to calling an ambulance in an emergency, but if the patient's state is critical, it is important to have an idea of their wishes for end-of-life care to avoid unwanted hospitalization and futile intervention. Ambulance paramedics are trained to respect such wishes and may advise on means of keeping the patient comfortable until death. However, if there is doubt about the patient's wishes and there is no clear documentation, paramedics may feel obliged to transfer a patient to hospital. While some people might think of a hospital as a peaceful place to die, the nature of busy emergency departments is such that tests and interventions are often set into motion very quickly, to the unending regret of loved ones, and a modern hospital is far from peaceful.

Everyone fears dying in distress. In our communities, with access to robust oncology, palliative care and other medical support services, we are able to reassure our patients that this can be avoided. I would advise talking to your oncologist, family doctor, and the palliative-care team about the things you or your family fear most. Having an open conversation allays many fears.

Key Points

- Pain and other troublesome symptoms at the final phase of life are readily manageable with modern means.
- A peaceful death can happen at home, in a hospice or a hospital, but it helps to articulate your wishes in an advance care directive.
- It's okay to openly discuss your fears to ensure appropriate counselling and timely management of symptoms.
- Involve your family in these discussions as they too probably share your worry silently.

32

The Impact of Being a Carer

The waiting room is full of patients today, and as I cast my eyes on the waiting crowd, I spot Leila sitting in a wheelchair. 'I will see you soon,' I signal to her husband Asif with my eyes. He nods gratefully at me.

When I call the couple in, I watch as Asif disengages the brakes of the wheelchair and prepares to wheel Leila in. She leans heavily towards one side and nearly loses her balance. He stops and carefully steadies her body. Displeased at something, she mutters a few words to him. He stops, pats her gently on the shoulder, and resumes pushing. At the entrance to my door, she says, 'I wish everyone would stop treating me like I'm breakable. I'm sick of it, really sick of it.'

Asif takes a deep breath. 'Alright, just let me get you in and I'll stop. I'm sorry.'

'It's okay,' she grumbles, as he parks her in front of my desk and takes a seat next to her. I feel a wave of sympathy for Asif, who looks weary and thinner than when we last met. His hair has greyed and his face is haggard; he looks like he could do with a hot meal and a long sleep.

Leila was diagnosed with cancer several years ago when she was busy with a full-time job and the task of bringing up their two late-teen children. She coped with the initial chemotherapy very well and even continued to work and drive the children to their activities. Asif had been expecting a much greater degree of upheaval and was pleasantly surprised at how smoothly things worked out. Leila remained well for nearly ten years before she developed a recurrence. This time, she felt sick from the start, and despite aggressive treatment, headed into a slow but progressive decline over eighteen months. Two months ago she developed brain metastases and the deterioration has been pronounced. She has lost the ability to walk and her vision is failing. She experiences headaches, has become irritable and has a disrupted sleep–wake cycle.

Following his wife's decline, Asif has been progressively reducing his working hours but had to stop working completely in the last six months. I know that his generous leave allowance ran out and now he is on unpaid leave. Their two children live away from home to be closer to work. They are supportive and spend some nights with their parents but their commitments vary by the week, making it difficult to rely on them.

When the nurse takes away Leila to monitor her weight and dress a small cut on her hand, I have a chance to be alone with Asif.

'How are you? You look unwell yourself, if I can say so.'

'People say I look almost as sick as Leila,' he jokes weakly. 'Maybe I am.'

'This is tougher than any job you have ever done,' I tell him. 'Leila is certainly becoming more dependent on your care, isn't she? You are doing a great job.'

He nods gratefully and I suspect he doesn't hear any praise for his truly remarkable work. Nudging the door shut, he opens up. 'I am completely exhausted. All day, I look after Leila's needs and try to keep up with the housework when she sleeps. At night, I sleep with one eye open because she is restless and often calls out for me.' Self-consciously, he adds, 'But doctor, don't get me wrong. I want to do this. It's what I always promised myself.'

'Would you consider admitting her to a hospice so that you could have a break?'

'Never,' he says emphatically. 'I wouldn't know what to do with myself if she wasn't home. My whole day is built around her and as I said, it's what I promised.'

We review his supports, amongst them a palliative-care nurse and his brother and sister-in-law who live nearby. He also shares that his finances are becoming precarious after they lost first Leila's income some years ago and then his in the last few months. 'We are managing and I know that I'll return to work one day. I tell Leila we are just fine, but honestly, it's unsettling to use up our savings. I worry about being poor.'

'When was the last time you went out alone?'

'Eighteen months ago, the day she found out the cancer was back. How can I forget that day?'

'How can I help you?' I ask, feeling overwhelmed by his situation. 'You have so much on your plate.'

'Nothing more, doctor. I'm just thankful that you appreciate what I am doing.'

Leila returns and after a brief chat, Asif wheels her out.

'Can I start pushing now?' he asks gently, obviously sensitive to her needs.

'I wouldn't be here without him,' she says, tears springing to her eyes. 'He is my rock, but I just wish things weren't so hard for him.'

Asif's eyes meet mine wordlessly as if to say, 'See what I mean?'

The population is ageing and more elderly people are being treated for cancer. Their carers are also older and troubled by their own illnesses. There is a greater pressure on hospital beds, but a hospital stay is often not restful, so it's understandable that cancer patients want to spend most of their time at home. This has great implications for the primary caregiver. You may be ageing or adolescent, a spouse or family member, or someone close to the patient.

How did you assume your role? Was it always going to be this way or did you find yourself edged into it due to circumstances? I recently met a patient's best friend who took over her care when her elderly parents suffered a nervous breakdown at their daughter's state. 'I felt there was no other way. Her parents practically brought me up – now it's my turn to help them.' Hardly anybody prepares to take on this role, but like cancer itself, people deal with the cards they have been dealt.

'I'm not doing much. She is the one fighting the disease,' a carer once said to me. Please don't underestimate the value of your contribution, which cannot really be matched by anyone else. Caregivers find themselves responsible for not only physical assistance but also emotional and financial support. On any given day, you have probably found yourself helping your loved one with cutting up a meal, assisting with showering, reading a book aloud, helping with a walk outdoors or a drive to the doctor, discussing troublesome symptoms, planning the future and managing the bill payments. Household tasks can be tiring and emotional tasks intense. If you feel exhausted, depressed or overwhelmed, you are like most carers.

Studies show that between 25 and 50 per cent of caregivers experience anxiety and depression; regrettably, most will not seek treatment due to their greater concern for the cancer patient. You may also be feeling socially isolated because you don't have time to go out and you're not as flexible as in the past. You become disconnected from friends and colleagues that you would normally debrief, and your life seems to exist in a cocoon.

Many carers who used to be physically active and understand the importance of staying fit report that they simply don't have a chance to get out. You probably find that fatigue prevents you from exercising, or maybe you lack the time after taking care of everything else. Many caregivers notice their diminished stamina after months of caring.

There is also a great economic cost to being a caregiver. The patient is often unable to earn and the caregiver needs to reduce hours, utilize leave or sometimes quit work altogether. Some caregivers resign in order to not exert pressure on their workplace. Many families use their savings or superannuation as a buffer. Cancer care is costly. Even when care is government-funded, patients rapidly accumulate out-of-pocket medical costs. Of course, the usual expenses don't necessarily slow down – the children's activities, grocery bills, electricity and water, the occasional takeaway meal. Caregivers frequently sigh that under the guise of managing money confidently they struggle with worries about the future.

Deeply personal stress, physical fatigue, lack of sleep, lack of exercise, financial cost – who would want to be a caregiver? The truth is that there are lots of you out there; lots of compassionate, conscientious people who willingly put their interests on hold to look after the sick. You would never name it so, but the silent sacrifice you make is inspirational.

If you are a caregiver, what are some of the ways in which you can help yourself? First of all, acknowledge that it's normal to feel overwhelmed, because the task is overwhelming. If you are feeling alone, make a list of people who might help you. Don't make excuses for them, just jot down how you think they might help. Perhaps someone could sit with the patient while you go out for fresh air once or twice a week. Maybe someone wouldn't mind doing your groceries or ferrying the children back from school. Could someone fold the clothing, put away your dishes, or cook some meals to freeze? I know these sound like small tasks, but remember that someone still has to do them, and if you can delegate some tasks, you can spend more quality time with the patient. Many sympathetic onlookers are eager to do something practical to help but don't know how to ask – give them a list of your needs and let them choose. I have spoken to many such volunteers who feel glad to be of use.

Confident caregivers may have better coping skills but in order to become confident you may need help. Sometimes this is in the form of practical training – learning to administer an injection, shower a patient, dress a wound or change a colostomy bag. Find someone to show you.

Some caregivers feel comfortable with their skills but need psychological help or counselling to address the bigger picture. They need to accept change, come to terms with grief, loss and guilt. Some caregivers need to learn how to manage anger, denial or other new emotions that surface in the patient. They find themselves unwittingly in conflict with the patient and are unsure about how to handle it. If you find yourself in these shoes, consider seeing a counsellor who can help you with some strategies. You may object to the time spent away from the patient, but consider that in the longer term, this will bring more quality to your interactions and help you as well. Sometimes a health professional may suggest that the caregiver and patient work on issues jointly to get the best result – it's worth giving this a thought, especially if there are deep unresolved issues that are likely to keep coming up. These days there is more than one way of getting help. If face-to-face meetings are not your style, you can try online or phone-based services as well as good reading resources that a cancer professional can recommend. Some caregivers find solace from joining a cancer support group, but others don't, or simply don't have the time for it. You know yourself best – do what helps you.

Amidst all of this, it is vital that you don't ignore your own illnesses. Make sure that you see your doctor to get your usual health checks, prescriptions and vaccinations. Mention your stress to the doctor and see if there are any ways in which she can help that you have not thought of.

Look after your diet, exercise and rest as best as you can, because when a caregiver falls ill things can change dramatically for the patient. Speak to the patient's oncologist from time to time to share your progress.

I speak to many caregivers in the aftermath of a patient's death. In my experience, the most content caregivers are those who felt positive about their engagement with the patient and that they had given the job their all. I want to emphasize that this doesn't mean they had an untroubled existence, or that they didn't have the occasional strong disagreement with the patient. It also doesn't mean that they didn't get tired and cranky themselves. In fact, the best caregivers are those who recognize that there is sometimes a limit to their own goodwill, and their capacity for sleep deprivation. But a common theme is that they found ways of communicating well and regularly with the patient and ironed out their differences, misunderstandings and expectations. One lady told me that when it was time to arrange her husband's funeral she felt he was guiding her through it because they had talked at length about his wishes. Another husband said that his wife had emphasized to him and the children that they had done everything possible for her comfort and this helped them cope with their feelings of guilt.

Finding just one or two common things that unite you and the patient is useful. For some people, it's prayer. For others, it's listening to a favourite song or reading quietly. Not all caregiver duties have to be about crossing off items on a list – sometimes, just being with the patient in the moment is the best way to demonstrate care.

I wish I could say that all the stress will disappear when you are no longer needed as a caregiver. But we know that the effects of being immersed in this all-consuming task are long-lasting. Many caregivers struggle with loneliness, guilt, anger and other suppressed emotions into the future. There are also enduring practical effects such as loss of income, sale of a house, or strained relations with friends and family. Regrettably, much of the work of recovery requires your initiative and advocacy and no one can blame you for being too exhausted to seek more help. However, help is available and it can make a difference to your future. So after giving yourself some time to recover, do go out in search of normality.

Perhaps the message I can leave you with is that as a caregiver, it's wise to anticipate some of the issues we have discussed and deal with them pre-emptively. They will help you cope better, and any time you cope better, the people around you, most importantly the patient, benefit. Don't worry about being selfish. You know that with all the heart and soul you have put into being a caregiver, your loved one would never want you to suffer.

Key Points

- Being a carer for a cancer patient is a highly stressful task. It is largely unrecognized.
- It is normal to cycle through many different emotions including anger, sadness and frustration as a carer. It is normal to want to take a break or get away completely.
- Anticipate the emotional, physical and financial cost of being a carer and actively try to build resilience and a support system by asking your doctor and local council. A specific cancer carers' support group may help you.
- Accept help from others without feeling diminished in your role. Speak to palliative-care services, a social worker and your council for practical assistance that is available for you.

Afterword

If you or someone close to you has suffered from cancer, I am sure you have asked yourself more than once, 'Why me?' This is a question that troubles and even haunts many people. After all, many of us adopt regrettable habits at some point, including smoking and drinking excessively, and many face stresses of various kinds. On the other hand, you might have led an exemplary life, driven by a significant family history of cancer or your own belief in living well. But such people also develop cancer. So it seems unfair to blame everything on a particular habit or one source of stress.

The fact is that cancer is not your fault. The fault is in your genes. Imagine your cells undergoing constant replication, where one cell divides into two. Normally, this process is carried out faithfully, in that each cell behaves as it is meant to. If a cell replicates incorrectly, the body has a number of internal safeguard mechanisms whereby the faulty cell is automatically destroyed and you don't even know it. Your organs continue to function normally. But every so often, an error happens. One error does not lead to cancer, but when genetic mishaps align, a cancer is born. Given the complexity of the human body, the remarkable thing is that cancers are not triggered more often – for this we have our internal safety mechanisms to thank. So here is the thing – cancer is unpredictable. It is a random event. And the longer you live, the more times your cells replicate, the more likely it is that things will go wrong by chance. Cancer is the flipside of our longevity.

By all means, you can eat well, exercise often, avoid known carcinogens such as cigarettes, and watch other triggers. But the evidence that these things definitely protect against cancer is not robust. Of course this does not mean that you should abandon healthy living.

For example, we know that smoking is harmful in a variety of ways. Smokers who don't develop cancer still suffer from a range of serious health problems that can be just as onerous. Similarly, persistent stress should be managed not because you fear cancer but because stress has the ability to deeply affect so many other aspects of our life.

So what I am saying is that if you are feeling betrayed by your body, or questioning why cancer happened to you, take heart. In a life of random events, you have been unlucky. I don't think I meet anyone who is not shaken by a cancer diagnosis, but the people who can put it in perspective are the ones who cope better. They treat it as part of the large scheme of life that is not easy to understand and even harder to control, and then they focus on the practical aspects that they can control. So they try to be actively involved in decision making, in deciding when to take a holiday, when to give up toxic treatment, and how to spend their free time well. They strive to maintain some enjoyable interactions. I want to be absolutely clear that I am not suggesting these people never suffer angst, doubt or dismay – of course they do, but they work through these emotions, realizing the importance of maintaining a positive outlook on life.

'How can I be positive when I am dying?' a disgruntled patient once asked me. I thought it was a great question. Few things are more irritating than a cancer patient being told to buck up or to just try a little harder to get over things. It is downright galling for people to be told that their cancer is the golden opportunity they needed to value the gift of life. If you care about someone with cancer, my advice is to support him quietly rather than by making such grand statements, even if they are well-intentioned. As another patient observed, 'I resent being reminded that were it not for my cancer I wouldn't have made peace with my brother. No one knows what I might have thought as time passed.'

Returning to the matter of being positive – I don't claim to have a perfect answer, but in listening to patients young and old, who are fighting the shock and the setbacks of having cancer, I find some universal themes amongst patients and carers.

Acceptance is one. They accept that this is a random, unlucky event that they will deal with as best they can. Being reasonable is another. They adjust their expectations with the course of the disease. This means that plans need to be made and cancelled at short notice. By plans I don't only refer to major occasions but simple everyday activities like lunch, a walk in the park, and seeing a friend, which have to be adjusted according to how you feel.

Working through fear is another important theme. Notice I don't use the term 'conquering fear', because from what I see, fear of cancer and its consequences does not just vanish one day. It is an ever-present and live issue whose impact changes with the disease. People who accept fear as a normal emotion, articulate it and look for explanations to mitigate it are the ones who process fear successfully. For example, if you are afraid of a particular experience occurring during chemotherapy, talking to your oncologist may help you realize that it is unlikely in your case, and that may be all you need to address your fear. If you are fearful of voicing unintended thoughts should you become confused, talk to a palliative-care professional about ways to manage this.

Religion and spirituality feature largely in many people's lives. A patient once asked me if she should reclaim religion in her illness because nothing else made her feel better. Her devout parents felt ambivalent about this, she said, because the move was self-serving. Another patient was a lifelong atheist who said that he found comfort in adhering to his views.

Many patients are sustained by their religion, philosophy and spirituality. By spirituality, I'm referring to the search for purpose and meaning in life. Spirituality may be heightened at the closing phase of life, when people wonder whether there is a deeper meaning to life, whether suffering has a reason and whether your experience is part of a larger, unknowable scheme. Religion, on the other hand, provides people with a structure for thinking about some of these questions. Each religion provides guidelines or a code of beliefs and behaviour based on its beliefs.

Some people find familiar customs comforting when coping with difficult news and for nourishing hope in the longer term. For others, the sense of community and the practical consolation or answers that their religion provides are all-important. Religious beliefs feature strongly in people's decisions about cancer, as well as in coping with the dying process. Some people believe that religious or spiritual patients cope better with the dying process because their religion gives them an explanation for death. A spiritual person may experience less emotional distress because there is a framework for regarding death not as a personal failing but a normal part of the cycle. However, it has also been observed that highly religious patients may feel more conflicted about dying and may want everything done to preserve life even when aggressive measure may be associated with harm. Some of this may be explained by the belief in a religious miracle or the fact the religion creates connections that patients want to hold on to. Sometimes religion and spirituality create anguish when there are no good answers. Of course, none of these explanations is absolute – studying the religious and spiritual beliefs of cancer patients is not an exact science. But while detailed arguments about religion are not within my remit, I do think that having an anchor in life is vital. This doesn't just apply to cancer patients but to human beings in general. At the least, an anchor protects you from drifting. It also allows you to regard your life with purpose. And whether your purpose is to finish the woodwork in your garage or to serve God until your last breath, what matters is having purpose itself. So if religion brings you purpose, by all means embrace it.

If you do not have a strong faith or religious background, you are not alone in our diverse, multicultural society. Probably a good half of my patients do not specifically nominate seeking solace in religion. What seems a universal human need, however, is to feel connected. Even patients who are very ill and unable to socialize express the need to feel connected to their close friends and family. Having people care about their welfare and express concern for it allows patients to retain dignity. Therefore, I would strongly advocate that you build such connections in your life and encourage existing ones. This can be tricky if people equate connectedness with incessant physical and emotional interaction because the truth is that when you are spending much of your energy facing cancer it isn't easy to nurture social relationships. But we are social beings and a good anchor for many patients is human company. Don't worry, you will discover a level of engagement with others that suits you. In keeping with the theme of this book, I would encourage you to do what feels right for you.

As you read this, you may be facing a new diagnosis, in the midst of treatment, in remission or contemplating terminal illness. You may be the beneficiary of modern advances and be a cancer survivor. All these phases of your cancer experience are associated with particular concerns. No matter what, I hope that in reading this book you have discovered facts, practical advice and consolation to help you navigate your experience. Remember that there is no single correct response to the many situations that will arise along the way. But there is a correct approach, and that is to be involved in your care, listen to your gut instinct and make decisions that suit you. I wish you luck.

Acknowledgements

This is the most cherished of my writings but also in some ways the most difficult, for it has taken me a great leap of faith to believe that my humble counsel might inform the deliberations and choices of those who have to navigate a feared illness like cancer. I owe a mountain of debt to all those who have nurtured my aspiration to get me to this point.

My parents, Kaushal and Urmila, and my brother Rajesh, with their enduring love, are a wellspring of inspiration. I also thank Taru, Sankalp, Shreya and Sneha for their encouragement. The blessings of my extended family in India are never far from me.

The Week's Stanley Thomas and Sridevi took me on as a health columnist ten years ago. Their loyal support has been instrumental in my development as a writer. They have allowed me the privilege of communicating with Indians from all walks of life whose questions and comments informed this book. I find this both poignant and fitting.

While writing this book, I have met doctors and nurses who have worked tirelessly, and mostly without recognition, to honour a strong commitment to helping underserved Indian patients. I salute them and am proud to add a drop to their ocean of work.

Rukmini Chawla Kumar of HarperCollins has been simply wonderful to work with. I admire her sound sense of the needs and sensitivities of Indian cancer patients and her diligent efforts to bring this book to life.

I have undiluted pleasure in acknowledging the school that shaped me. Mount Carmel School in Bhagalpur, Bihar, was a modest school with unforgettable teachers. We had few resources but dreamed large. I remember the patience with which Miss Ruby held my hand and taught me how to write. I remember the pleasure with which Mrs Leena

Sahay read my earliest writings and brought order to my ideas. Mrs Shakuntala Sinha, Mr M.M. Jha and Mr S.K Jha, Miss Susan Nanda and Mrs Pramila Agrawal are others who had an enduring influence on me. No words can do justice to the personal pride they took in seeing their students prosper – it really was the greatest catalyst for success.

The philosopher Euripides observed that life has no blessing like a prudent friend. My Indian upbringing was and has remained rich in friendships. I am particularly grateful to Swati, Jyoti, Reena, Divya and Jaya for their unalloyed affection and unfailing belief in me. I know that I would be a lesser person without them.

To my dear husband, Declan, I owe thanks for seeing this book in me long before I ever did. Anjali, Sachin and Rohan, my treasured children, I love you for creating the cheerful and noisy spaces within which I write, although you sometimes accidentally manage to delete my writing! Yet no book would be complete without you, so thank you for being so patient again while I finished being an author.

Medicine is a wonderful vocation and one of the true privileges of being an oncologist is to repeatedly witness the very best of human nature. I am humbled by the willingness of my own seriously ill patients and many people, including those in India, whom I have never even met to share their concerns and advice, uplifting stories and accumulated wisdom so as to ease the journey of others. I know that their selflessness will provide sound advice and gentle solace to all those who find themselves tossed about by a diagnosis of cancer. To these silent, compassionate and courageous contributors, I owe my greatest thanks.